Power

Tales of Being Dead Last

JOHANNA OUTLAW

ISBN:1545570906
ISBN-13:978-1545570906

DEDICATION

This book is for all of those who finish last at every race. We truly get the most out of our registration fee. Those who have their own police escort as they are the last one to finish. Those who take the full time that a race course will give you. We may be slow but we don't give up. Just like the turtle, slow and steady to the finish line.

CONTENTS

ACKNOWLEDGMENTS

I would like to thank my parents, Rev. and Mrs. Frederick Outlaw, my siblings Rashida Outlaw and Ahmed Outlaw. I would like to thank my best friend, the drill sergeant, my number one zero who put the idea in my head to write a book, Gregory "tall drink" Clanton.

I would like to give a special thanks to all the groups who have played a part in my career as an athlete, NCRC Women's beginner running group, Capital RunWalk Fit-Tastic, Raleigh Galloway, the nOg run Club, BGR Raleigh and last but certainly not least Tri It for Life.

CHAPTER 1 - 2008

I was introduced to the world of running purely by chance. I was attending a weekly TOPS (Taking off pounds sensibly) weight loss support group, meeting during the summer of 2008. I noticed the writing on a polo shirt that a fellow TOPS member was wearing that read NCRC (North Carolina Roadrunners Club) Women's Beginner Running Program. I asked the young lady wearing the shirt about it. She told me it was a local running program for women.

My inner geek went home directly after the meeting and searched for the program online. Lo and behold I found out the program was starting soon and registration was open for the upcoming season. I paid the registration fee. I attended the information session at a local community center. I was nervous and excited. I had never run before outside of PE class in high school. This would be a brand-new chapter for me. I was ready for the challenge. The information session went over the program. It is a 12-week couch to 5K program that prepares women for running their first 5K race. The goal race is Women's Distance Festival in September. There was a young lady who spoke about her previous experience with the program and how it helped her lose weight. I immediately identified with her because she was black. I kept thinking to myself if she can do it, I know I can. Her name is Rhonda Logan. We have been friends ever since.

The first run was scheduled for Saturday July 26 at Shelley Lake. I can remember that day like it was yesterday. I was nervous and excited which is typical I have discovered over the years before any race or training session. The group was broken into pace groups. As I had never run outside of PE class I opted for the very last group. Each group is partnered up with volunteers. No one runs alone. It is a no drop group. YEAH!! I am partnered up with the AMAZING Jean Hagen-Johnson. The goal is to do about 1.25 mile. The distance around Shelley is about 2 miles. Jean has us doing a 1:1 interval. Run for 1 minute and walk for 1 minute. After the first few intervals, I am breathing hard. Jean slows the interval down to 30s:1 minute. That works for me. We make our way around Shelley. We come up on a slight incline. OMG!! I think I'm going to die. Jean tells me to take a rest and get my heartrate down. Then we start up again. We pass groups of runners on the trail. They all know Jean. She yells out to one lady runner she knows and asks her how much is she running today. The lady responds, "only 8 miles" As I am barely making it through the 1.25 miles, this chick is out doing "only 8 miles" Jesus be a fence. I later discover that she is part of the Raleigh Galloway group, a marathon and half-marathon training group. We make it back around to the other side of Shelley. I opt to walk up the sidewalk that runs parallel to Millbrook because my car is parked close to the entrance. Jean heads back to the parking lot. I have completed my very first run. I discover later that my entire body is completely sore from head to toe. It took me an entire week to recover. I came back the very next Saturday. When I couldn't make, the Saturday runs, I would get out on my own.

The target race for the program was the NCRC Women's Distance Festival held on September 27, 2008. I signed up to do the race. The race was held at Halifax Community Center in Raleigh. My finish time was 1:18:53 with a pace of 25:33.

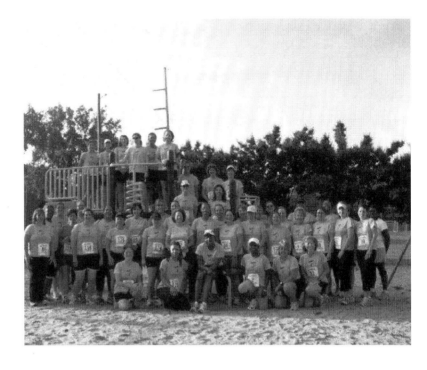

After completing the Women's Distance Festival race, I opted to get more involved with the run club. I started volunteering at races that the run club sponsored. I got a chance to see what a race looks like from the volunteer perspective. You really learn to appreciate all the work that goes into putting on a race.

The next year I was sidelined with a knee injury and was unable to do any running or walking. I continued to volunteer at races. In 2010, I came back to volunteer with the women's group. After a conversation, I had with Rhonda we both decided to sign up for our first half-marathon, Rock 'N Roll Las Vegas.

CHAPTER 2 - 2010

The Magnificent Mile

The Magnificent Mile is a mile-long race held in Raleigh, North Carolina on September 19, 2010. The race was founded by Sarah Witt, a former marathoner, who is diagnosed with Primary Lateral Sclerosis, a motor neuron disease related to ALS or Lou Gehrig's disease.

As a member of the NCRC Women's Beginner Running group, I decided to run the Mag Mile with my fellow beginner runners as a warm-up to our target race Women's Distance Festival the next weekend. I figured I would step it up a notch and decided to register for the competitive race just to see what my time would be.

Race day arrived on a gorgeous, warm and slightly humid Sunday afternoon. As we prepared for the start of the race, I felt apprehensive that I may or may not make it through one teensy mile. As the race started with the onlookers cheering on us, I knew I could make it to the finish line. I ran and walked the mile through downtown Raleigh, my personal drill sergeant and friend Rhonda Logan, ran the course alongside me on the sidewalks. As we headed towards the finish line, ladies from the running group who had finished met me and crossed the finish line with me. That meant more than words can say. My finish time was 16:15. I was in shock and amazement when I saw the time because it felt like I had been running FOREVER.

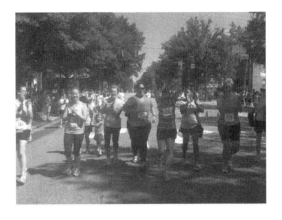

Rock N Roll Las Vegas Update: I was dragging my feet about registering, training and making travel arrangements. Rhonda was much more determined than I was. She had booked a flight and a hotel. She was in the game. I was on the bench watching the game. Rhonda went to Vegas in November and ran her first half-marathon that year.

2011

When 2011 started, I decided to give running another try. I found a Couch 2 5K program online. I was committed to the program for about 2 weeks and then I fell off the training wagon.

CHAPTER 3 - 2012

St. Timothy's Spring Sprint

April 21, 2012

I have been on a journey to become a runner since my participating in the 2008 NCRC Women's Beginner Running Program. Practice makes perfect. I decided to participate in my 1st 5K race/walk for the year with the annual St. Timothy's Spring Sprint. I registered as a competitive participant but I was always planning to walk the course as I am starting my runner journey again. I had the pleasure of walking the course with a good friend Sevanne Moushegian and her mother Rita Selmont. Of course, I am a slow walker so I was bringing up the rear. Little did I know I would have a race stalker AKA the police car that was following the end of the participants. At the 2-mile mark, he decided to leave me but he did leave me with the route so I could make it back to the finish line. I was very appreciative of this action. When the cop left me, he passed Sevanne and her mom who were a little ahead of me. She was very worried wondering where I was and the cop told her we were doing less than 18-minute mile so we would be on our own. I finished the course in 1:07:37.

Fit-Tastic Spring 2012

2012 was the year I decided to get serious about running. I signed up for Fit-Tastic, a local couch to 5K training program sponsored by Capital Run Walk, a local running store in Raleigh. Guess who else was signed up? You guessed it, my partner in crime Rhonda Logan. The group met twice a week for group runs. It was a 12-week program that ran from March-June. The target race was Susan G Komen race for the cure in June.

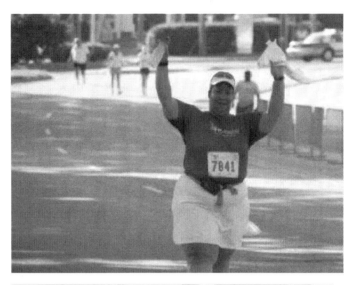

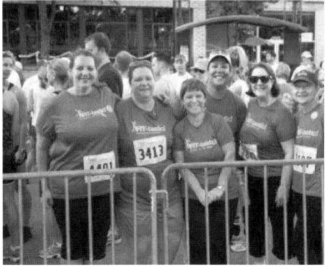

During the 12 weeks, Rhonda and I got to talking about venturing into half marathons. She had done 1. I had done 0. We were both talking about signing up for the Raleigh Galloway Marathon and Half-marathon training program. This time I was ready to get in the game.

Raleigh Galloway Program Summer/Fall 2012 Training program

I attended the information session for the Galloway program. I was completely sold on the program and that I could complete a half marathon. I was so hooked, I went ahead and signed up right there and paid the $159 registration fee. I was in it to win it.

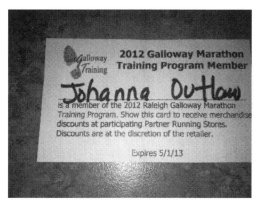

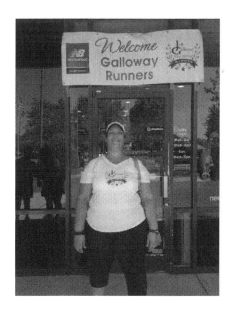

The Mag Mile

September 2012

During the summer of 2012, I signed up again as a participant with the NCRC Women's beginner running program. I continue my journey to become a consistent runner. The group participated in the Magnificent Mile race as a practice race before our target race a few weeks later. I enjoy the 1-mile distance, it is my favorite of all race distances.

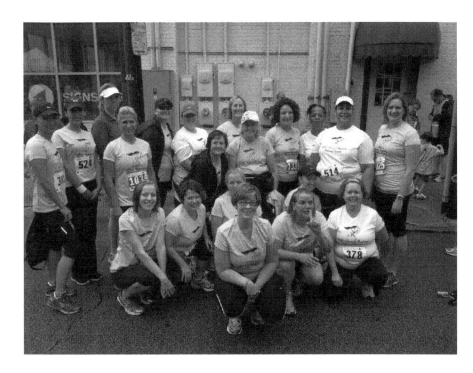

Monster Dash 5K

October 28, 2012

Raleigh, NC

On October 28, 2012, the annual Monster Dash 5K was held at Cameron Village. This race was the target race for the Fall season of Fit-Tastic, a run to walk training program sponsored by Capital Run Walk. This day I pulled double duty as a volunteer and a participant. I started feeling overwhelmed after rushing from my volunteer post to rush to my car to get ready for the race start.

Mother Nature decided to not allow Hurricane Sandy to not affect the race. The weather was overcast and cool in the 50's. This was great race weather conditions. I was just happy that it didn't rain. I am not a fan of rainy races.

After taking a group photo with my fellow Fit-Tastic peeps, I headed to the start line. Because I am a slow runner/walker I headed to the very back of the start line. I was very happy to see there was a stroller group participating in the race. There was even one stroller dressed up as Darth Vader.

At 2pm, the race started up Clark Avenue. Having done the course route a few weeks before as part of Fit-Tastic, I knew to walk up Clark Avenue because it started up a hill. Once we turned on Oberlin, I keep my pace slow and steady. I love going down Oberlin because my church is located there. It felt so good walking past there. Too bad my church family wasn't there cheering me on. After I made the turnaround and crossed over Wade Avenue, I was joined by none other than Rebecca Sitton who helped through the rest of the course. Once we turned down on Clark towards the finish line, I decided to run down that infamous hill. To my surprise, I finished with a new PR of 1:00:40, woo hoo! On to my next race.

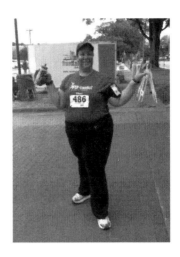

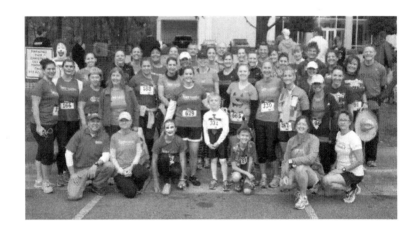

18

Raleigh City of Oak Marathon & Rex Healthcare Half-Marathon

November 4, 2012

Raleigh, North Carolina

A few years ago, I decided at some point I would like to do a half-marathon. To accomplish this goal, I joined the Raleigh Galloway Training program back in May. I started off with good intentions with Galloway, ran with them for 3 runs. I was sidelined with an injury that took me off training for 2 months. Before my injury, I signed up the Rex Healthcare half-marathon with about 5 and half months to train.

Once my podiatrist cleared me to start running again, I start back to training with the goal of my first half. The morning of November 4 arrives with a low temperature of 40 degrees and about 30 % chance of precipitation. I arrive at the race site about an hour before the race starts with first half jitters. I run into NCRC & Galloway peeps. This helps to settle some of the jitters. After I put my fleece in my bag for the bag cheek, I really feel how COLD it is outside. I wonder did I wear the right running clothes.

I line up with the 3:00 hour pace group lead by Brad Broyles and Barbara Latta. I knew already this was a very high goal but I would give it the old college try. As 7am nears, I realize this is it, this is what I have been waiting on for since the week after Memorial Day. 7am arrives and the gun goes off and the race begins. I start off slow and steady and we make it to the start line about 5 minutes after the race start. It feels so great seeing all the spectators along the start rooting us on. I keep thinking to myself I am really a runner. We head down Hillsborough street and I'm reminded of a Fit-Tastic run that ended with me running in the rain for the first time. Then I start running out of gas and start walking. By this time, I have lost the pace group and my fellow Galloway member I met earlier at the race. I keep my pace slow and steady. We turn down Ashe Avenue and this is very familiar ground to me so I decide to run down until we hit Western. Then my personal stalker AKA Raleigh finest Paula O'Neal pulls up beside me and gives me the spill about hitting the sidewalk. I check

19

the iPhone and I'm at 20:00/min pace. I keep it moving. As I head up Boylan, my very good friend Rhonda Logan is walking towards me as she is a course monitor for the race. It feels so great to see a friendly face. About mile 4, my body needs a restroom and thankfully there is one at the water stop. At mile 5 an angel named Rebecca Sitton meets me and she walks with me the rest of the way. As we approach mile 6 which is Clark Avenue which is completely uphill, I am hurting bad. My left hand is swollen like sausages, my feet are hurting and I am feeling slight dose of hypothermia. I decide that I have gone as far as I can. I push through to make it back to Hillsborough because even though I haven't made it to 13.1 I still want to cross the finish line. I slowly make the final distance down Hillsborough to the finish line. I look up at the clock and it reads 2:50 but I know it's not my real finish time because I am missing about 6 miles. I have still gone further than I have ever gone in a race. I am extremely proud of that accomplishment.

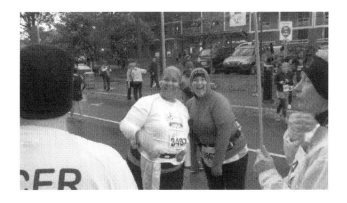

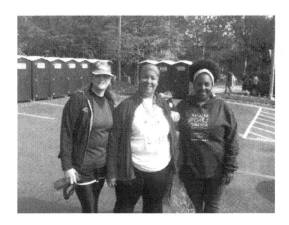

CHAPTER 4 - 2013

St. Timothy's Spring Sprint

April 6, 2013

Raleigh, North Carolina

The St. Timothy's Spring Sprint was held on April 6, 2013 on the campus of St. Timothy and the North Hills community. The race proceeds benefit the Rotary Club's Styres Scholarship Fund and WakeMed Children's Diabetes & Endocrinology. This was my third time participating in the race. I registered as a recreational participant.

The morning of the race the temperatures were in the 60's with a cool breeze. Due to the cooler than normal April temps, I opted for long sleeves and long bottoms. I had recruited a few like-minded friends to participate in the race as well. At 9:30am the race started down Rowan street. As I have learned about any race that is held in North Hills, it does have its name for a reason. That reason is there are nothing but hills in North Hills. We lined up not quite in the rear as we should. Our pace started off much faster than we had been training. We were still dead last which is where the fun is. As usual I was followed by own personal stalker Raleigh's finest, the police. I noticed as we came up on the country club we were coming in from a different direction. The race course had changed from 2012. I truly believe they added more hills if that was possible. My motto is slow and steady until you finish unless there is a snatch and grab van that pulls up to tell you that you are under pace. Sorry about that, that was a DIVAS flashback. I really enjoyed the race this year. The course monitors and the water stops all stayed staffed until I was finishing. My 1st time participating in this race, they had all vanished by the time I had made the turnaround. I see my email from 2009 has made a difference. Back to the story, as I approach Rowan Street I have never been so excited to go up another hill. I know this is my LAST one because I am making the final trek to the finish line. As the last one to cross, the MC for the race asks me how I feel. I responded "GREAT" The finish is my favorite part of the race.

Divas Half Marathon

April 2013

North Myrtle Beach, South Carolina

After the City of Oaks DNF, I was motivated to reach my goal of completing a half marathon. I signed up to do the Diva North Myrtle Beach half marathon. If you know me, you know that I LOVE the beach. Going to the beach to do a race is right up my alley. Initially there was 4 of us planning to do the race. Due to a family emergency, our trip was down to 3. We left for Myrtle on Friday with the race being on Sunday morning. We checked into our hotel and then headed to Broadway at the beach for some dinner at Planet Hollywood. On Saturday, we ate breakfast at one of the best spots in North Myrtle, the golden griddle pancake house. After a hearty breakfast, we headed to the race expo. After the expo, we hit the outlets. You can't go to the beach and not go to the outlets. After stimulating the economy at the outlets, we head back to the hotel. We relax in the hotel and then head out for an early dinner.

Sunday morning arrives and we are up early and getting ready for the race. My friend Sharon Mincey meets us at our hotel and scoops us up. We head over to the race start. It's about zero dark thirty at the race start. Race starts at 7:30am. Michelle Blank and I are walking the race. We line up in the back. After all the runners take off, we take off. I hear a spectator say, "you can walk this race?" I'm thinking to myself you sure can. The race is described as walker-friendly. What I was soon to learn was yes, it is walker friendly but you need to be a speed walker lol.

Michelle has taken off; her pace is much faster than mine. I'm just moving along at my normal pace. I notice there are 2 ladies behind me. They are snapping pictures along the race course. At mile 2, my bladder decides it needs to be emptied. I see no porta johns. I pass course monitors and I ask if there is a port a john. They have no idea. I keep pushing. I have just passed mile 4 and I am coming up on a water stop. It's nothing but sistahs. They are cheering and yelling at me. They are very encouraging. As I get closer, they ask me what I need. I'm like I've been waiting for 2

23

miles to use the restroom. They point directly to it. I finally get to clean out my bladder. As I am contemplating my decision to do this race, I hear a truck pull up. I swear fore God that it sounds like they are about to pick up the porta john. I hear some ladies yell out, "there is someone in there". I finish my business and yes, the utility guys are out there picking up traffic cones and about to pick up the porta john that I was just in. I get back on the course and try to re-adjust my clothes. I have probably gone about .10 of a mile and out of nowhere I see this white van pulled up beside me. I immediately think if this is a snatch and grab, all I have is my iPhone and $20 but they are welcome to it. The van pulls up and a lady tells me that she must pick me up, she's the race SAG wagon. Apparently, I am below the required 16:00/minute pace and I must be picked up. Dip me in axle grease and call me slick. (that's a Cars reference). I am being picked up by the SAG which I would like to call the snatch and grab van. I am feeling completely disappointed that this is happening. I have been consistently training and felt I was ready to do this. The race volunteer tells me that they have a timetable of where runners must be at certain mileage on the course. They need to open the roads back up. We keep riding and we pick up the 2 ladies that I saw earlier. These 2 ladies are Jennifer Bailey who is now Jennifer Davis and Julia Chaffin. They are from Charlotte. They are members of a triathlon group called Tri It For Life. We became Facebook friends. We take pictures in the SAG wagon. We are making the most of the situation. We are all discussing the time requirement situation. They tell the SAG wagon driver you are going to have a van full of folks. As we keep going on the course, we pick up more ladies. We even pick up Michelle who was moving at a good pace. We pick up another lady from Charlotte named Kristina Blake. Some of the Charlotte ladies mention she is going to be disappointed because she had been working so hard to get ready for the race. We are riding for a while. Everyone is bummed that we are in the SAG wagon. Then the driver stops further up on the course, maybe mile 7 I think. She lets us all out. She tells us we can keep going on the course but if we fall under the time she will pick us up again. Another option is to cut across and head to the finish line. Yes, this is technically cheating for those who stick to the rules folks out there. At this point, Michelle and I get out the van and we take the easy way out. Yes, we cheated. We still had another mile and some change left to get to the finish line. We are on that final stretch on ocean boulevard. We pass by the tiara and feather boa station. We get a tiara and a feather boa. We make that final right turn onto main street and we cross the finish line. Technically this is my 2nd DNF but I maneuvered my way onto the finish line to get a medal that I did not earn. A part of me felt bad once the shirtless firemen handed me my medal. I did not earn it. I did pay for it with my race registration. I went ahead and took the medal. I posed for finish line photos. Deep in my heart it did not feel like a true victory. What I learned from this 2nd attempt at a half marathon is that I must not quit until I complete the entire 13.1 miles.

8th Annual Gateway Outer Banks marathon weekend

Southern fried half marathon

November 10, 2013

I travelled to the OBX for the first time in 2012 with friends who were participating in the race. I thought it was so cool they received 3 medals for doing the challenge. I decided to sign up for the 5K and half-marathon challenge with some friends.

The 8th annual Gateway Outer Banks marathon weekend was held on November 8-10, 2013. We were up at 5am to be at the race for 7am start. We took the shuttle from Nags Head Elementary to a block from the start. I dropped my gear bag off at the drop off. What I have learned for me I need to have a pair of flops or slides to change into IMMEDIATELY after a race or a training run. I head back over to the start and they are lining up the corals

Just about ALL of Galloway that I saw was in Corral F for FABULOUS. I realized on Saturday that I left my Gymboss in Raleigh so I figured I would hang with my pace leader Robert Shanks. About 7:15am Corral F starts off for 13.1 miles from Nags Head to Manteo. Wouldn't you know it I need to go potty and we have just started. I'm on the course with 2 of my Galloway peeps, Robert Shanks & George

Weinstein. We stick with 30/30 intervals. I'm doing good until about mile 2 and I hit the porta potty. My calves/shins start kicking up but I kept pushing through. I enjoyed going through the neighborhoods. The second neighborhood we run into a dog minus his owner. He's friendly and didn't bother us. George runs ahead of us after we make another potty stop. Bert takes of ahead of me. Now it's just me myself and I. I just keep moving one foot in front of the other. Marathon runners are passing me by. I get back to 158 and slowly make my way to the bridge.

The bridge OMG the bridge from HE-double hockey sticks. I slowly take my time and I only stop twice. Once I make it the bottom I check my iPhone and it's still has juice. iPhone 5C Rocks!! I also stop at the aid station because I really must GO. As I go, I'm saying a prayer to get me through to the end. I am making my way to Manteo and I'm so excited. I know I have less than 3 miles to go. I keep thinking I just did that on yesterday so I can do it. Mile 11 comes up. I'm thinking only 2.1 miles left to go. I see mile 12 and I'm thinking I only have 1.1 miles to go. OMG why was the last mile the hardest. I keep pushing through. The spectators are cheering me on "you're almost there". One of OSBE bikers yells out "you got this I saw you at the 5K yesterday". Every little bit helps so I keep chugging along and I'm making my way into the heat of Manteo and going through the neighborhoods and folks are outside their houses yelling "you're almost there" "only 2 more turns". Then this one guy who I've never met in my life walks up to me and say, "inch by inch to the finish." He has white and blue pom poms, how did he know that's my school colors. I make the first turn and then I make the last turn. I can see the finish. I can hear the music. I hear "sexy and I know it". I start dancing to the finish line and I'm so emotional when I cross the finish line in 5:04:47. OBX finisher!!! Up next jingle bell run on December 7 and myrtle beach half in February 2014.

CHAPTER 5 - 2014

Tri It For Life

As we were travelling back from the Outer Banks, registration opened for the 2014 season of Tri It For Life. I was signed up as an athlete to train for my first triathlon. TIFL is a women's only couch to sprint triathlon training program that was started in 2006 in Charlotte, North Carolina. I participated in the Raleigh chapter. It is a 12-week training program. Athletes are coached by mentors who are ladies who have completed at least one triathlon. We meet 4 times a week to swim, bike and run. There are brick trainings involved as well that include doing 2 of the sports back to back.

The beginning of my TRI journey

Sunday February 23 marked the beginning of TIFL (Tri It For Life) training season with the Raleigh chapter. Sundays are swim training days. This was also FIT FEST. That means athletes will be able to try on TRI gear that they can order for the upcoming Ramblin Rose on May 18 or for upcoming training sessions. Being a fluffy girl, I'm always "concerned" about sizes. When it came my turn to try on, I ask about the larger sizes and they did not have any available. I was given sage advice of heading to local athletic/sports/running stores i.e. REI, Dick's, Fleet Feet or Inside Out. My experience with Dick's and their non-existent plus size section is not good. I won't even waste my time. I will call the other stores before I get in the Max to see if they have the available sizes I'm looking for. The geek in me went and asked google. I LOVE google. Google rocks. Google directed me to an old fav site of mine that was a go-to for running gear years ago, Junonia. They have tri suits in "real" plus sizes. The prices are $$. I wasn't sure what a tri suit will cost. OMG this sport is expensive.

We met at TAC (Triangle Aquatic Center) in Cary at 1pm. Swim was from 2-3. Part of the requirement for TIFL with swimming is you MUST wear a sports bra under your swimsuit. Initially I thought that was odd. After several laps in the pool, I totally get why it is a requirement. First drill involved floating and kicking while holding onto the kick board for 8 laps. Yes, I said 8. This was not my favorite drill. It didn't matter how much I kicked I felt like I was not moving anywhere. I used my left arm for freestyle stroke and then I was booking. Laps were cut down to 4. thank goodness. Second drill involved going down one lane with 1 arm raised and kicking from the hips. this drill proved to me a lot better. I discovered one side is easier than the other. This drill was also for 8 laps. It was cut down for 4 laps. HALLELUJAH. The last drill was 3 strokes and then come up on your side for 8 laps. This was my far my FAV. I got so caught up I was doing 5 strokes and overworking myself :-). Then it was cool down time. This involved going down the lane with freestyle and coming back with elementary backstroke. I love floating on my back or swimming. I was more concentrated with my arms and not moving my legs. 1 of my fellow TIFL beginner swimmers came behind me and said, "kick your legs" She even started moving my legs for me. Which caused me to laugh and spitting up water. I crack my own self up sometimes.

Then it was quitting time. Everyone else started getting out the pool on the ledge. I was determined to do the same. This was quite a feat. It took AWHILE. After several hundred attempts I finally got up on the first ledge and after another hundred attempts I got up on the final ledge. I literally laid there on my back. I told someone "just bring my car to me right here".

I survived my first TIFL swim training. A day later every muscle is talking back to me. I know it's a good thing. It's what happens every time I do some form of exercise I have not done in a long time. I am TRIing this TRI thing. :-)

St. Paddy's Run Green Kilt Run

March 2014

Raleigh, North Carolina

I love supporting local races. I have signed up for St Paddy's Run Green kilt run. Race starts at 2pm. Since its downtown, I know to head there EARLY around 12. I must not have been the only who had that same idea. Because traffic was heavy. I could get into the parking deck on Blount right across from Marbles, SCORE. I had no idea that deck went to 7 levels. I was on level 5. I run into a few NCRC peeps, Galloway peeps and TIFL peeps. We really do all run in the same places. We line up for the kilt run around 1:30pm. The line was HUMONGOUS. They are checking kilts, belts and buckles and taking the release form. Then we line up in the starting corral. People are still coming in. I am thinking they have a good chance of beating the record. I heard today they had 1455 kilts runners short of the record of 1700. Race starts about 2:15. It's 200 meters which is 2 turns around Moore Square and we're done. People are running like they have $$ on this race. I take my time as it just 2 blocks. We make the final turn towards the finish line and I love my time it's about 3 minutes. I shall call it a PR :-)

After leaving the race, I am on an official mission to acquire a bicycle as this is a very necessary tool to complete a triathlon. I have been told about 2 local bike shops in the area, All Star Bike and Performance Bike. I heard to the All-Star bike shop on falls of the Neuse.

Mock Tri = official TRIATHLETE

April 27, 2014

Raleigh, North Carolina

Today was the mock Tri. What is a mock Tri? It's a practice of the triathlon race on the same course without timing and full TIFL mentor support. Now, I would like to give a shout out to group 2 and its awesome mentors Amy Funderburk and Melva Peed.

I never sleep well the night before a race. Last night was no difference, tossed and turned all night. Kept thinking about the race. My hands go to sleep continuous through the night :-(I woke up once and it was 3:45am. I knew I still had more time to sleep. Back to sleep. By the time my alarm went off at 6 I was still tired. I am so not a morning person but I make it work. The car and bike are already loaded. All I needed was to fill my filtration bottles. I decided to put ice in my camelback, smart thinking my young patoine (shout out to my fellow Star Wars fans who got that). I'm in my Tri suit getting ready and I'm already seating. WTF?? I decide at the last minute to grab a t-shirt to wear over my Tri suit. Once I get to AE Finley I literally hits me like a ton of bricks it's cold as ice outside. My body temp was up so I didn't really feel it. Fellow TIFL athletes are there and setting up their bike and transition area. I can hear "Let's get it started in here" in my head. SN: I love the black-eyed peas, even paid some serious $$ to see them at PNC.

I'm told I'm with group 2. We are at the back of the outdoor pool. I realize this Y has it going it. What do you expect it? This is north Raleigh, home of big $$$$. I pass some of my Fit-Tastic peeps Claudia & Penny. I finally find the number 2. I pull in next Melva. Little did I know she would be my rock that would get me through the day.

I start unloading my bike and someone tells me to go check in. I grab my $10 and head to the registration table. I run into my buddy Julie Reed. She has that "what did you get me into Jo" look on her face. I get that look a lot because I am a good motivator to talk folks into doing stuff.

As I am in line to register and check-in, I see one of my running and NCRC buddies Rebecca Sitton. She has come out to root us on. She is a triathlete herself. I'm listing my emergency contacts. I always put down my mom. I mention that they may not be able to find her since she's in Florida on vacation. Amy tells me to list someone who is local in the event I get hit by a car. OUCH! I understand the need. I put down tall drink. Who is tall drink? Tall drink is a very good friend of mine. Tall drink is my nickname for him because he's a tall drink of water. My nickname is BIG BABY. He is the only one who can call me that. We've known each other for almost 14 years. He's like the big brother I've never had. Whodini song is in my head "Friends, how many of us have them"

I head back to finish getting my transition area ready. I'm told that my towel is too big. On race day, I will have less space. I fold my towel to a much smaller size. This is what happens when you miss the transition clinic. I was in rock n roll 3.5-hour recovery nap. Umm hmm that was some good sleep. A few of us head over to potty before we get ready for the race. I hear someone yell out "you know it's a race because there's a line to use the bathroom" The difference is we have real bathrooms and not porta potties. I'm so glad I went because my nerves have kicked and that's all I'm going to say about that before it really gets to be TMI. We head over for the swim. We start the swim in group order. Our group is 2nd. 250 yards of swimming any way you can. That's what I'm talking about. Up and down. Up and down until the ladder. Some of my fellow TIFL athletes pass the ladder. Overachievers :-)

We wait on the rest of our group. For some people, the swim is the hardest. For me the hard part is the next sport, the bike. After the swim, we head back to transition and get ready for the bike. Then we walk our bikes up to the bike start. Cross over the speed bump and we are off for the 9-mile bike ride.

We head out of the Y and onto Baileywick, slight downhill. I'm thinking we must come back up this hill to reach the finish. We are down by Baileywick park and turn into the neighborhoods. This part I know. Turn and turn. Hill and hill. I remember pretty much walking my bike up most of the bigger hills. We get to a turn of a super busy intersection. I believe it was Mt Vernon Church Road. This is a 2-lane road. Cars are booking on this road. Cycling on a busy road with cars is a scary experience. There's a slight uphill and I ride too far on the right and hit the grass and I take that as sign that I'm supposed to walk my bike. Melva and I walk our bikes up. Melva tells me "2 fingers to walk the bike" this is a good tip. We make it up the hill. 1 down a billion to go. We ride some more and then we turn left back into the neighborhood. Ride and ride we go. We hit another hill and I'm so tired and spent I think of Cartman from South Park "screw you guys I'm going home" is running through my head. Emotions hit me hard as I'm struggling and I get off my bike and I break down. My rock AKA TIFL mentor Melva comes over and talks to me and ask me "if we need Jesus" I tell her yes. Then I think about the story of the kid who was kidnapped and was singing so much that the kidnappers brought him back. I tell Melva yep I so can see that happening with my 2 youngest nephews. Braylon Jamal Outlaw would be asking for some food and a smartphone to play with. We start singing the song that little boy was singing "Every praise is to our god" we only hum the chorus. it gets me back into the riding groove. I continue to push through. We make it to Carrington AKA the devil. Amy mentions that downhill is where I rock. I go out 2nd. Down Carrington "fly like the wind bullseye". Downhill I love. It's the uphill where I have issues. I attempt to bike up but I'm so tired that I just say FU and walk up Carrington. My group is waiting for me at the top. Amy tells we have a few more turns and then we will be headed back to the finish. I love that word. Few more turns and we are riding across the bridge over 540. I know it's literally 2 more turns. We get to the stop sign. I see TIFL mentor Alicia at the entrance to the park. We cross Baileywick. We regroup and then head back to the Y. I struggle up Baileywick. There's another hill. Hills how I hate you, let me count the ways. I walk the bike and then I hit an intersection and I can feel that I'm starting to break down again just like mile 8 at myrtle. I drink some water and get my breathing under control. Melva says "come on you have to ride in for the finish" I get back on the back, cross Baileywick and head towards the finish. The course monitors tell us to dismount before we hit the speed bump. Dismount and walk the bikes back to the transition area. I drop the bike. I stop RunKeeper and commence to take a selfie. Melva and Amy are yelling at me "you don't have time for selfies" I'm thinking to myself there's always time for selfies. They rattle on about being timed during transition. All I hear is the teacher on Charlie Brown talking to me ROFLMAO.

I'm 2/3 done with the TRI. We head out for the last 1/3 the 2-mile run. At this point it is see a familiar face. He yells out "you got this" slow and steady through loop 1. At the water stop I see "the boy" AKA Trish's son. I talk to him about RNR. He tells me he finished in 3:00 then corrects himself and tells me it was 2:58 :-)

We finish loop 1 and who is waiting at the entrance of the Y, tall drink. He rocks. We are headed back in for loop 2. a TIFL mentor walks up to me and tells me "you and I were lined up together at City of Oaks" I respond "yeah back in 2012" She tells me "you got this" Loop 2 here we go. I'm doing ok except that I'm tired and my lower back which is my problem child is aching like no tomorrow. We are making our last turn and we see TIFL mentor Brittany. She gets a call I'm assuming from the finish line and they are asking about us. She lets them know we are headed to the finish. We turn on Baileywick and then we are at the entrance to the Y and headed to the finish line. Everyone is there waiting for me to cross. I absolutely love they are cheering and yelling. It feels so good to cross the finish line. I cross the finish line. Trish walks over to me and tells me "You are a Triathlete" Yes, I am now a triathlete. I see some of my Group 2. High fives are going all around.

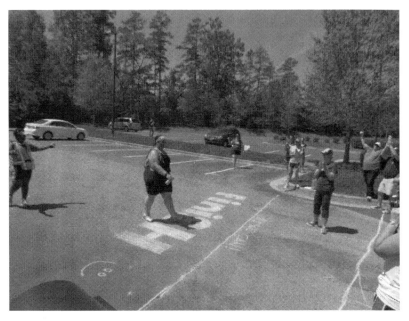

I notice the merchandise table is being broken down. I was ready to go shopping. Guess I should have done that before the race but I was holding out. Then it's group picture time. I love a group picture.

Then I realize I still must walk all the way back to my car and oh joy load it up. Who cares? I have finished my first mock tri and I am now a triathlete.

A few things I need to work on: nutrition (barbecue lodge night before a TRI is not the way to go), strengthen lower back muscles, as much hill training I can get in in the next 3 weeks.

T minus 3 weeks until the real kahuna, Ramblin Rose May 18.

I would be remised if I didn't give a special shout out to my BFF Neti Jenkins and her crew for coming out to the picnic to support me.

Ramblin' Rose Raleigh

May 18, 2014

Raleigh, North Carolina

I've been training for the last 12 weeks in preparation for completing my first official triathlon. That day was May 18. The race consisted of 225-yard swim, 9-mile bike and 2-mile run. Race was held at AE Finley YMCA in Raleigh.

My plan was to be at the race site at 6am to get a good parking spot and a good spot in the transition area. I realized I was super-duper early when the race was still being set up. Early bird gets a good parking spot and bonus an end spot on the bike rack. This was my first TRI so I was kind of wandering around like a lost kid in the mall. A lot of my TIFL mentors would come up to me and guide me on what to do. I love those chicks. Helen Bac AKA Claudio Mello help me mount my bike properly and all the way to the end of the rack. Martha helped me attach my timing chip. Then I headed over to the orange shirts aka the volunteers to get marked. I was familiar with being marked as we went through the same process during the mock TRI. I made my necessary pre-race potty stop. Went back to the transition area to get ready for the fun.

I met up with the 3 amigos. Let me explain the 3 amigos = myself, Julia Reed and Erin Keener. We head over to the front of the Y for the pre-race announcements and the start of the race. After the announcements, our TIFL cheerleader Sharon lead us into our TIFL cheer. Who are we? Triathletes What do we do? Finish Strong. We were so loud they could probably hear us in Durham.

We filed into the Y. We line up in the gym based on swim ability. 10 is the

35

fastest level and goes down to 1. I signed up with group 6 along with Julie. Like most things, I got talked into moving up to group 7. Peer pressure I tell you.

Group 7 is headed towards the pool. I'm thinking OMG we are about to swim. We head towards the pool. Erin and Julie are ahead of me. Then I'm up next. I climb into the pool and start swimming. I'm moving slow and steady. Next thing I know I'm apparently holding up traffic because there are like 3-4 women who pass me. No problem. I'm in no hurry. At the end of each lane I see a TIFL mentor who is calling my name and rooting me on. Then I'm on the last lane and TIFL mentor Amanda Law is pointing to the ladder and tells me "Jo you are done. You can get out" why do feet act like they can't move. I do make it out the pool. We head back to the transition area. There are spectators along the route rooting and cheering fellow participants are running past us to get to the transition area. Did I mention we noticed as we were getting out of the pool, we could see ladies already on the run course. That meant they had already done the 9-mile bike course. Holy Smokes batman.

I make it to the transition area. I'm wishing I had brought a shirt to put in over my Tri suit but I totally didn't think about that when I was packing. Shoes and socks are on. Camelback is on. Helmet and gloves are on. I drink some PowerAde and head out for the bike run. I meet up with other 2 amigos. We head out round 2. This is my 3rd time on this course so I know it very well.

I'm rolling down Baileywick and cross into the neighborhood and I see folks headed back. Rebecca Sitton yells out "good job Jo" I see my fellow TIFL Emily hauling tail back to the Y. This bike course is not for the faint. It is up and down. Up and down. We hit mount Vernon which is a busy road and when we get to the hill.

We all walk it along with everyone else. We get to the top and get back on. Turn and turn through the neighborhood. Then we make that right-on Country wood. I know what's next the devil disguised as Carrington. I rock downhill. I will pass you going so fast it will make your head spin. I'm hauling down Carrington. Then here comes the uphill. I don't even try, I get off the bike and walk it up. Because there is no shame in walking. After that it really is just a few more turns back to Baileywick. When I ride over the bridge and see 540 I am so excited because I know soon as I will be headed back to the Y. I'm head down the hill and I see the turn and the cops and course monitor are holding traffic and that turn is made with ease. I have less than 1/2 mile to go. I pedal and pedal. I see 1 of the amigos Julie I'm front of me. She is walking the last bit and I am still biking and I yell out "on your left" then there's the turn into the Y. I see a. TIFL mentor and she yells out "you can dismount now" she tells the hard part is over.

I walked my bike back to the transition area. I see people leaving which means they are done. I hear someone yell my name and it's a friend of mine who has come out to see me at the race. That just made my day. I load the phone in the armband, take the helmet and gloves. Then I head out for the 2-mile run. The run at this point is a slow stroll. Slow and steady until the finish. It felt so good to cross that finish line and see all my TIFL ladies waiting for me as I crossed. I am a triathlete.

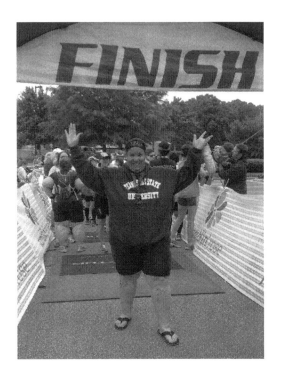

Gigi's Cupcakes 5K

October 18, 2014

Raleigh, North Carolina

This was the inaugural race for Gigi's Cupcakes of Brier Creek. I first saw the race advertised on Facebook. The appeal for the race was the $25 entrance fee includes an official race shirt, a medal AKA BLING and a Gigi's cupcake. Who wouldn't do this race? Bonus it's a 5K only 3.1 miles.

Ever since I got into triathlons back in January/February of this year I have "lost" my running mojo. Crazy, right? What can I say, I rather ride 13.1 miles on my bike than run 13.1 miles in a half-marathon. The mojo must still be in me because I am already registered for 2 ½ marathons in 2015.

The race was held on Saturday October 18, 2014 in Brier Creek in Raleigh. Race start time was 8am. The race coordinator sent out an email on Thursday to give race day information. Email stated park near Target or the movie theater. The race will start in front of BJ's. I came in from 540 and took the Lumley exit and came in right by BJ's but I saw no indication of a race. I'm keeping an open mind since this is their first race. I drive towards the Movie Theater and park there. I see one of my TIFL sisters is already there. My energy level is increasing. We meet up with the rest of our TIFL comrades.

There are a few announcements about the race but I can't make out what the guy is saying. Thankfully someone could interpret for us. The start of the race is now in front of Target. We walk towards Target. I get a text from a friend asking me "is the start at BJ's or Target" There was a little confusion on the race start location.

We are lined up in front of the Target. We head back to towards Gigi's where the actual "start" is. I somehow have lined up in the middle of the race and runners are taking off fast. I have learned from previous races don't get caught up with the fast take off because I won't make it past mile 1.

We cross the timing mat at the start, I see the wonderful finisher's medals. Then we turn left towards Brier Creek Parkway which is a slight hill. It's Raleigh there are hills everywhere. We turn left on Brier Creek Parkway. They have 1 lane blocked off with cones for the race, very nice. The race turns left into the Brierdale shopping center. We pass by Earth Fare and then exit the shopping center. We cross over Lumley and we turn left onto Arco Corporate drive which runs behind Brier Creek shopping center. I've noticed that I have my own personal escort following me on the course. As we head towards the end of corporate drive he pulls and tells me "you have a bit of downhill ahead of you". We make what I will call the 2nd to last turn on the service road that runs parallel to 70 and you can see the wonderful uphill that is left. Then I make the last left back into Brier Creek shopping center. A few of the course monitors are walking behind me. Suddenly, the DJ is riding behind us taking music requests. One of the course monitors tells me "you're almost there" I really am because I see the finish line. As I get closer to the finish line, 2 ladies come up to me and run to the finish line with me. Random acts of kindness can be found if you are the last one to finish a race. As I cross the finish line, one of the finish line volunteers walks up to me and hands me a card. It dawns on me they have run out of medals. I have heard this can happen but this is the FIRST time it has ever happen to me. I'm still trying to optimistic since this is their first race. In the back of my mind, I'm

40

disappointed. I'm started to feel overheated all sudden and go find a chair to sit in. Some of my TIFL sisters call me to the finish line to take some pictures. One of my TIFL sisters Melissa Yergey Daly, I shall call her ANGEL walks up to me and asks, "where is my medal?" I tell her they ran out. Do you know what she did? She gave me hers. She told me I earned it and she has plenty of them at home. That's what you call LOVE. My official finish time was 01:04:41. I'll take it.

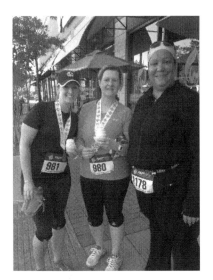

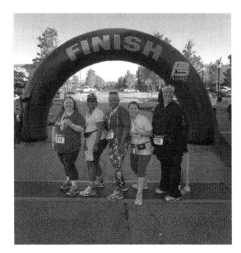

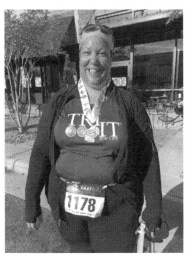

CHAPTER 6 - 2015

First TRI of 2015

Lifetime Fitness Indoor Triathlon

January 3, 2015

Cary, North Carolina

FOMO fear of missing out. I truly have that :-). If one of my TIFL sisters post in our Facebook group about any type of race, tri or any event that is going on. I always feel that I should participate. If not for the health benefits alone. If there is BLING involved I am in. I saw a post about Lifetime Indoor TRI and everyone was signing up, of course I signed up as well. Cost was $25 and you get a shirt. Not bad at all. The other 2 triathlons I have done cost around $80-90. This was a huge drop in price. The indoor TRI was January 4, 2015, 1st Sunday of the new year. About a few days before the TRI, emails were sent out confirming your wavenumber and start. I hadn't gotten any email. I was starting to worry that maybe I didn't register. I went to the registration page and was in the process of registering when I clicked on my account and saw the receipt for my registration, mystery solved. 1 of my TIFL sisters saw my name in her wave so she knew I was registered. I was still dealing with cold that I had been self-medicating with for a few weeks. I knew the TRI was going to be a semi-struggle because I haven't done any real form of exercise or training and my body was recovering from the cold.

Saturday night I started getting my gear together. Since this was an indoor TRI

43

I didn't need my bike or bucket, woo hoo!! I have a new swim bag that I was going to use. I pretty much had all my gear together and headed to bed. I woke up Sunday morning excited and nervous. I headed to Lifetime Fitness-Cary. I was there about 9:50am. As I am heading into the gym, I hear someone call my name. It's one of TIFL/Fit-Tastic/Galloway buddies Claudia. She tells me "I knew I recognized that car with all those bumper stickers". My car could never be the getaway car because it is not inconspicuous at all lol.

We head into the gym. The lady at the front desk tells us to head down the hall to the TRI check-in desk. I pick up my race bib, swim cap and race shirt. We head to the lockers. We run into other TIFL sisters who are already there. A few of us are members of another TRI group, Black Triathlete Association. We take a few group pics with our new BTA shirts.

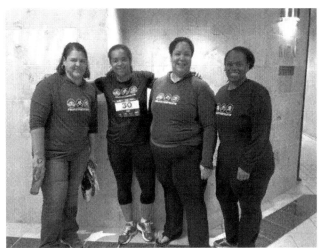

It's about time for me to get ready to swim. I head out to the pool. Sharon Johnson tells me "Jo you should go for the lane by the door so when you're done you are right by the steps". Good advice. Tina Alexander and I are in lane 1. At 10:40 we start our 10 minutes in the pool. I don't know what it is about the pool. Every time I get in, I am in love and I also feel like I have totally forgotten how to swim. Note to self: you need more pool time. I could tell I was struggling because every time I would breath when I went under the water it felt like I couldn't breathe. At one point, I just kept my head above water and just swam. It was kind of nerve wracking because I kept an eye on the clock so when it got close to 10 minutes I made it to the end of the lane and just waited until the counter was done because I was so done.

Swim is done, I have 10 minutes to transition from swim to cycle. Let's call this event #2, changing out of a wet sports bra to a dry sports bra. I truly believed the right girl felt like it was dislocated during this process. I head to the cycle studio. This is event #3, locker room is on the 1st floor, cycle studio is on the 3rd floor. I'm about done done when I get into the cycle studio. They have already started. I'm OK with that. One of the Lifetime trainers helps me get set up on the bike and get my feet in the clips. Lawd have mercy, my right foot is not working with me or the Lifetime trainer, takes us several tries to get it in there. I'm on the spin bike for the very first time. I wish it was over before it started. I pedal through the longest 28 minutes of my life. When we count down to 0 I was never so happy in my ENTIRE life. I shall call getting off the spin bike event #4, one leg was off and the other leg was still on. I am my very own comedy show and didn't even know it. I'm off the bike and headed to the cardio area for the final event, 20-minute run on the treadmill. My body is so sore from the bike, climbing down the steps is a real task. I meandered my way over to the treadmill. We line up by race number. since I'm 81, I'm in position #1. I tune my iPhone to DJ Kool genius playlist and I'm off. At this point I am not concerned about

45

running, I am just trying to get the feeling back into my arse and my feet. Slow and steady on the treadmill grooving to the music. This was my FAV event of the entire TRI. When the 20 minutes is over, I have completed my first TRI of 2015 and my first indoor TRI. I am a TRIATHLETE.

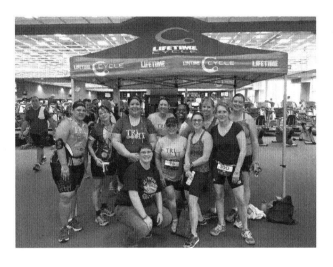

Charleston Shrimp & Grits 5K

January 17, 2015

A very good friend of mine, Sharon Johnson, chose to celebrate her birthday by having a girl's weekend in Charleston. I have a severe case of FOMO (fear of missing out) so I was in for the trip. Of course, there is a race involved. Charleston marathon weekend included 5K, half-marathon, full marathon and "recovery" bike ride. We opted for the 5K on Saturday and I opted for the 20-mile bike ride on Saturday.

The 5K is called Shrimp & Grits. When I read about the race I knew I was going to LOVE it. The race was on Saturday January 17, 2015 starting at 9am. We head out for the race around 8:15am. Per the GPS, we are about 10 minutes from the race start. We get to the high school where the race is being held. We find a good parking spot. As we start making our way to the start, I notice other runners have on different color race bibs. I mention it to my fellow weekend roommates. Sharon AKA the birthday girl walks over to the gear table and ask, "where is the 5K start?" The volunteer responds North Charleston. We look each other and realize we are at the wrong place. We hop back in the truck, put in the correct address and hit the road. We get to the 5K start at 8:45am.

We head to the race start and they have a coffee cart that is giving out FREE coffee. There is heater that a few runners are huddled by. About 8:58am, the race announcer makes a few announcements and then we are off. As we head towards the start line I spy green ribbons, blue ribbons and white ribbons on medals. I'm thinking to myself there is a medal for the 5K finishers, sweet.

I'm jamming to my old-school playlist and taking it one step at a time. This is only my 2nd time in Charleston so I am unfamiliar with the route. I just follow those in front of me. RunKeeper lady keeps counting down every 5 minutes, I'm moving at 20:00/mile pace. That is good since I haven't done a 5K since the fall. This is my first race post-stress fracture recovery. Mile 1 comes up right past a church. The route continues past a park and I past mile 2. We make our way back towards the start and I have met 2 fellow walkers who are Charleston natives. We hang through the rest of the race. The last mile has a slight incline. There's a mile marker for mile 22 which is right by a police course monitor. He jokes "you don't have 4 more miles to go" I'm thinking that mile marker could really mess with someone who isn't paying attention.

We head back towards the finish and past the back of the post-race party. Then I see Mile 3 marker. There really is 2 right turns left. I make that final right turn and I see the finish. As I cross the finish, a finish line volunteer walks up to me and hands me a medal. I LOVE bling!! First 5K of 2015 is in the books, finish time 01:10:14. ☺

Longest bike ride to date

January 18, 2015

Mt Pleasant, South Carolina

One of my awesome TIFL sisters planned a birthday weekend in Charleston. Of course, the weekend included a race but as part of the marathon weekend, they have an after-race bike ride. The bike ride has 20, 40 and 60-mile options. I opted for the 20-mile option. I still consider myself a newbie cyclist. We made a pit stop at performance bicycle on Friday and I walked around like a kid in a candy store. I need so many things for my bike. I know what my tax return or my STI aka bonus will be going towards just like it did last year when I bought my bike.

We get up Sunday and start preparing for the bike ride. I always ride with Camelback. I pulled it out my backpack and realized the reservoir top was missing. That's not good. I fill the reservoir up but water splashes right out. I'm thinking yeah this might be my first ride without the Camelback.

We load the bikes and our gear in the Jeep. We make a breakfast pit stop at Mickey D's. That egg white delight was delish.

We hit the road for Mt Pleasant. We miss our exit and then eventually get back on the correct route. Thanks GPS! We see a Charleston marathon truck at the entrance of our turn so we know we are at the right place. We see other cars with bikes so we really know we are at the right place. We had some location issues with Saturday's 5K.

49

After we park, we don't exactly know where to go for packet pickup. We assume it's in the building we see people walk to and from. SN: they need some signs. I pick up my packet and shirt. Bonus we got 2 shirts:1 for the 5K and 1 for the bike ride. As I'm waiting for Claudia and Sharon to get their packets, a lady walks up to me and ask, "are you with Tri It for Life" I'm like yeah, she tells me she recognizes me from the pics on the Facebook page. It's Raini Binnicker Kimball from TIFL-Charlotte who we were told was in Charleston for the same races. Her and her husband are both doing the 40-mile ride.

We chit chat a bit. Then we both make a very necessary pit stop to the facilities. I head out to get ready for the ride. I've decided to forgo the Camelback and tuck a bottle of water in my bag that's hitched to my bike. We take our bikes to the bike guy who's checking bikes. Bike is checked. 60 miles' riders have taken off. 40 milers are lining up, that's Claudia and Sharon. Then they are off. Last but certainly not least is the 20 milers that includes me, the 2 BTA ATL peeps we had dinner with last night. I see the TIFL Charlotte sisters have arrived. They were working on real CP time. The announcer talks to us about the route, rest stop and SAG support. At about 9:01am we are off. Every time I get on a bike I start to not like how big my bum is because it's always sore one second after I get on the bike. I have my cue sheet just in case I lose the group which I know I will.

We turn right out the school. We ride about 1.5 miles down and make a right on a main road that is flat but there's a bridge waiting for us. I try to ride up the bridge but my body tells me "Nah you should just walk" that's exactly what I do because there's no shame in walking. One bridge down, who knows how many to go.

Crossing this bridge reminds me of the bridge at OBX. At the bottom, turn right down another long road. I see a couple turn in front of me who I recognize are part of the bike ride. Then they make a left turn. I'm concerned that this is not the right turn. I pull off to confirm with my cue sheet and this is not the turn. I keep going straight. I see a road marking that confirms I was right. I keep riding and then I ride upon 2 female cyclists who look like they are having issues. I ask if I can help even though I really can't. They are happy that I stopped. They have it covered. I keep on down the road. My next turn comes up and it passes right by a church. I start humming "I need thee oh I need thee. At this point my quads are talking back to me, my upper arms are tired, my right foot keeps falling asleep and I'm freezing. Did I mention my nose has been running since I first hit the bridge? I keep riding and then come to a stop and I see green flags with the words "RACE OPS" and I'm thinking it's the rest stop. I turn into the gas station. I'm so excited. One of the TIFL Charlotte chicks tells me I'm a little early for the rest stop. You're supposed to be at 11 miles when you get there. They did the same thing, hit the rest stop twice. I'm just glad for a break from the bike for a few minutes. I enjoy the rest stop for a few minutes. Hit the facilities and head back on the correct route, I make a wrong turn and don't see the marking on the road. I head back to the main road and make a left. I see the road markings. I pass fort Sumter site and turn through the neighborhoods and make it back to the rest stop officially at this point. The SAG guy asks if I need a lift back, I really want to tell him YES but I want to push on through. The couple who made that "turn" ride in, I ask them about that. They tell me they were on the scenic route. I think we must go back towards the BRIDGE and the husband tells me no. I'm a little happy about that. The 3 of us head out and opt for sidewalks. There is a bridge but it's nothing like the first one. Did I mention there was some serious headwinds? Riding a bike plus strong headwind = frozen Johanna. As I make it down the bridge I see a sign that says, "welcome to mount pleasant" HALLELUJAH and thank you God we are back in the town we started in. I check my iPhone and it's in the single digits. I tell myself as soon as I hit 15 miles I'll connect it to the portable charger. I stop to do this and check my bag and you know what the charger and cable are not there. I realize they are in my gear bag which is in the jeep and the keys are with the owner on the 40-mile ride. I have no choice but to make it back because I can't call anyone and I don't know anyone's number by hard except the ride sag people on the cue sheet. I'm on the final stretch headed to the school and I just break down and cry because I'm ready to get off the bike, I don't want to ride anymore, I don't want to do any races anymore. I'm just sore tired and hungry. I see the turn for the school, there's a guy waiting there. He asks, "how many miles did you do" I reply 20 miles. He looks disappointed. I'm thinking to myself are you FU kidding me. I don't think about his reaction. I ride on to the parking lot. I disembark from the bike which takes 2 tries. I'm thinking I made it. I made it.19.1-mile bike ride is in the books.

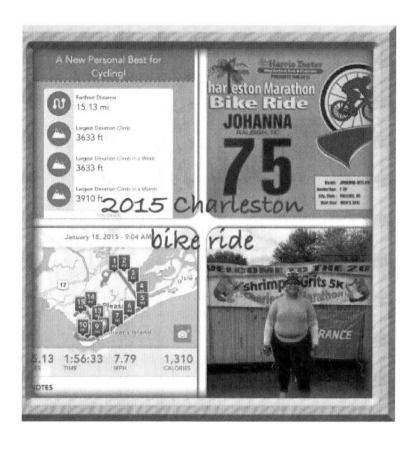

Shamrock weekend

March 20-22, 2015

Virginia Beach, Virginia

I turn 40 this year. I've been deciding on how to truly celebrate it. I decided to do races in cities I've never been. I heard of Shamrock from other runners. Then I got an email from the race sponsor, J&A Racing, about doing something great in 2015. It talked about fundraising with LIVESTRONG for the shamrock race. I put down $50 and I started fundraising as part of my race registration. I was committed to race $500. As of the week before the race, I have raised $800. I mentioned to a few of my TIFL sisters that I was doing shamrock and they decided to do it as well. We made it a weekend. As I read more about the race I found out there is a dolphin challenge of running the 8K on Saturday and the half marathon on Sunday. I contacted LIVESTRONG about changing my registration from the half to the challenge. They advised once I make my fundraising goal, my registration would change.

I rode up to Virginia Beach with Claudia and Tom Mello on Friday as Claudia and I were both doing the dolphin challenge. My fellow shamrock divas were only doing the 1/2.

Shamrock 8K

March 21, 2015

Saturday morning came and I headed to the shuttle at the hotel at 6:30am. The 8K didn't start until 7:45am but I wasn't familiar with where everything was. Early bird gets the worm. I drop my gear bag off and head back to the race. I hear someone talking to me from one of the hotels. I'm thinking "do I know this person" turns out it is one of TIFL sisters from Charlotte who I met at the Diva NMB race on the SAG wagon. She invites me back to her room to warm up because it's about 30ish degrees outside. Brr it's cold outside. I meet her other weekend roommates and Julie, another TIFL sister from Charlotte who I met on the SAG wagon at Divas in 2013. It might be true, I know a lot of people. You get around in this running/triathlon community.

Jen and I head to the start line. We are in corral 16 which was like a mile back from the start. We run into Angel and Tiffany from TIFL charlotte and Claudia and Tom Mello. It didn't dawn on me that we wouldn't start at 7:45 until they started moving the corrals. We didn't hit the start line until 8:25. Angel Tiffany and I walk together. We are in no hurry. Angel and I are doing the half tomorrow. Tiffany is 17 weeks pregnant, she's not trying to do anything fast and furious either. We notice we have our own personal escort, VA Beach sheriff behind us. KEWL beans. We notice all the food places as we walk down Atlantic avenue. Not a lot of them are open which is a good thing because we probably would have made a detour. We make the first turn onto the end of the boardwalk and we are hit immediately with a headwind.

55

The wind coming off the Atlantic Ocean is no joke. A lady walks up to us and tells us the SAG wagon told her "you need to catch up with the pacers". Isn't that something they called us the pacers. Do you know that same lady ended up passing us? Hilarious. We turn right at the end of the finish line chute. That sucks because you see the finishers headed to the party tent. We are back on Atlantic and there are people walking on the street with us and there's a car that tries to run us down. Dude yells out "there's a sidewalk" we yell back "we're in the race" IDIOTS. We pass a course monitor so apparently; the streets are not open. We tell him about the car and he can't believe it. That confirms we were in the right. We make the turn onto the boardwalk and make the final stretch towards the finish. OMG it really feels like the last green mile it's so long. I can see the finish line but it just seems so far away. A lady comes up to us, she's one of the race officials. They are about to start one of the kid's races. She's going to walk us to the finish line. This chick means business. "Make room we have 8K finishers coming through". We cross the finish line holding hands, Angel, Tiffany and me. My feet are screaming at me. All I want is my flip flops from my gear bag. 8K is done in 01:53:13 which beats my St Paddy's Run Green 8K time from 2 weeks ago, and that makes it a PR ladies and gentlemen. 1 race down, 1 to go.

Shamrock Half Marathon

March 22, 2015

Virginia Beach, Virginia

As every runner knows you don't sleep well the night before a race. I kept tossing and turning all night long thinking about my race day game plan. 5am wakeup call wakes us up along with everyone's cell phone alarm ringing. The shamrock divas are waking up and getting our race day gear on. Our plan is to head down to the shuttle at 6 and get to the race with plenty of time before race start. I go back and forth on wearing my TIFL hoodie because the forecast shows the temperature is in the 40s. I opt to wear the hoodie. We head to the lobby to catch the shuttle. The lobby is full of fellow runners who are waiting for the shuttle. I must give kudos to Wyndham because they have the shuttle system very organized. We are aboard the minivan AKA the shuttle. It takes us literally less than 5 minutes to get to our drop off spot which is 1 block from the race start.

This is Mary's first 1/2 so we are super excited for her. We snap pre-race pics by the start line. Then we head to the gear drop which is literally a mile away because we are in corral 12 the last one. We made a strategic decision to pack all our stuff in Mary's gear bag because she's the fastest off all of us and will be at the finish line first. Gear is dropped off. We join the lines for the porta potty. What I have learned is you must carry hand sanitizer when you race because you might need your own. That's all I'm going to say about that. The ladies have decided that we are going to join corral 8. Since I have a serious case of FOMO (fear of missing out) I join in with them. Corral 8 is up about 7:20am. We walk to the start line and everyone except this chick takes off running. I set the Garmin and opt to just walk the first mile and let me legs warm up.

I'm listening to my shamrock race playlist on my phone and I'm just enjoying the first few miles. A few people pass by giving my high fives and fist bumps. Mary Molly from Raleigh who I know from being in the same running groups passes me. Angel from TIFL charlotte passes me and asks me if I'm ok. I'm a lost at mile 2 so I'm ok. Then I hit mile 2 and my bladder starts to YELL at me. I see a porta potty over at a construction site. I made a pit stop. A lady yells "hey you all found her secret stop" pit stop is done. I get back on the course. One foot in front of the other, I'm headed towards mile 3 which is a major water stop. At this point, Rocketeer by Far East Movement is playing I'm in a good zone. I start dancing and waving my arms like a plane. I'm hoping this good zone lasts. One foot in front of the other. I opt to decide to just keep walking, no interval running. I'm on this long lonely road that looks like it's literally going nowhere and it curves to the left and there is an aid station with a band and they offer me a mimosa. I've never had an adult beverage while being on a race course. I only take a few sips and then throw it out. It warmed me up for a few minutes. I head into the entrance of Fort Story, a US naval base. I hit the 10K mark and I make sure I hit the timing mat. The volunteer laughs at me as I do it. I'm starting to feel a tender pain on my right foot. I'm thinking uh huh the toenail has broken off. I try to ignore it. Did I mention my feet started hurting about 2 miles back but I've gone numb to the pain? I'm just walking and jamming to my music apparently too loud because I missed the lead vehicle telling me to get out of the way because apparently, the lead male marathon finisher is coming through AKA the royal

Prince. Yes, I am hating because I am I'm the same race but I need to get out his way. Rant over. More marathoners are coming through. I'm really feeling like I should just call for a taxi or at least Lyft ride. Then I see this guy pass me on one of those bikes and I do a double take. This dude has no legs just arms and he's hauling tail down the course. I think to myself I seriously have no real reason to not finish since I have 2 good legs that are working. This buttercup sucked it up and kept on walking. I'm making my way out of the naval base and I've not noticed they have taken down the mile markers for the half but left up the ones for the full. I pass the coolest water stop on the planet. I see some of the kid volunteers have Popsicles. They ask me do I want one. Yes, I do. I take a blue one and it's like the best thing I've ever had in my entire life. The sun is coming out. It's slowly getting warm. I pass our hotel for a second time. If I wasn't such a bling chick I would have just went back to the room but wait I don't have a key Mary and Sharon do. Oh well I must make it to the finish. I pass marathoners who are heading on the course where I just left, poor things. I see 2 runners wearing NBMA (National Black Marathoners Association) shirt which is super cool. My boyfriend, Charles Leveringston, calls me and I tell him how tired I am and how my feet feel. He tells me to block it out and tell this race course I got it. I tell him to talk to me about anything to get my mind off the pain. He tells me he ate my box of caramel delight Girl Scout cookies. Yep that did it. Because I'm no longer thinking about the pain. I really don't care about the cookies. I just needed the distraction. He hangs up and Chrisette Michelle starts playing again and then my phone dies. Note to self: do not stream your music from iCloud while doing a half marathon because it will 1) kill your battery and 2) suck up your data usage. Even the geek has lessons to learn. No music and the Garmin has died as well. It's just my mind and my breathing keeping me company. I make that curve past the Cavalier, stop by the last water stop and drink water and Gatorade. Head down Atlantic, make that last left turn that brings me to the boardwalk. If this isn't the longest part. I can see the finish line in the distance but it seems so far away. Out of nowhere an ANGEL appears. Her name is Angel. She's my TIFL sister from charlotte who has been my rock my sword and shield all weekend. She's already finished, came back out to find me and walk me into the finish line. We post for the official race photos. We head into the last stretch of the finish line. People are cheering and I hear my name over the PA. I cross the finish line of my 2nd completed half marathon. All I want is my flip flops. Dolphin challenge is done. 18.1 miles in 2 days. Put a fork in me because I am DONE.

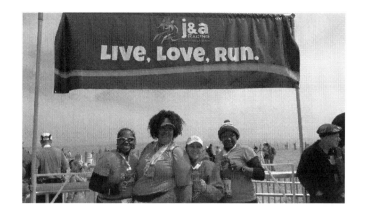

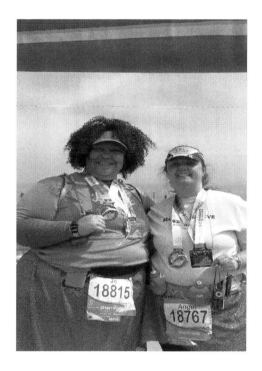

American Family Fitness Half Marathon

November 14, 2015

Richmond, Virginia

On November 14, 2015, I participated in half marathon #7 in Richmond, Virginia. I went into this race un properly trained. I have no real excuse for not training except I just didn't train. This was my first time doing this race. Since the beginning of 2015 I've been traveling with a few of my TRI sisters for race weekends. We started off with Charleston in January and finished off the year with Richmond. We drove up Friday afternoon and immediately hit the expo. I LOVE race expos. It's like Christmas morning as a kid except you are your own Santa Claus. I didn't get too caught up. I only bought 4 pairs of Balega socks (they were buy 3 get 1 free) and a pair of 13.1 earrings. I did score a free race shirt from the All-American marathon which is held down in Fayetteville. I remember some of my Fit-Tastic peeps ran it last year.

I'm often told that I know a lot of people. People fail to realize I've been around this running community since 2008. I'm alumni of a few running groups, i.e. NCRC Women's beginner running group, Fit-Tastic, Raleigh Galloway, a one-time appearance at lifetime run and of course last but certainly not least Tri It For Life.

We check into the hotel. We decide to find some food at the hotel. The reality of race day is starting to hit me emotionally. I have a slight breakdown at dinner. What can I say I'm an emotional chick. Our hotel is 5 blocks from the start. We decide to sleep in until 6am and head over to the start around 7am.

Saturday morning shows up in like 5 minutes. Seriously it was just that fast.

It's about 39 degrees outside. I'm from Alabama and that's cold to this southern gal. I'm glad I packed my jacket and almost thought about rolling with my hoodie but my clothing is not disposable so I left the hoodie in the suitcase.

We pick up a quick bite from the hotel. We make our way to the rave start. Lord have mercy nobody mentioned the HILLS we had to climb from the hotel to the rave start. By the time, we made it to the rave start I'm already sweating. Mary asked me "jo are you sweating already" I'm like I was born sweating. That was the pre-race workout. We see the start line. There are people everywhere. Race day excitement is in the air. All 4 of us are in corral K but we pull a "Sharon" and line up with corral H. I don't know why because all the corrals are going to pass me by anyway. I'm a team player, sometimes. I see a few familiar faces from Raleigh. Carolyn Quarterman is in our coral. She tells me she has done the full before but not the half. Larry Stroud from Galloway finds me and we take a pre-race picture. I met Larry at a Galloway training run at Capital Run Walk in 2014. He came up to me after the run and told me you kept going out there and that's all that matters. I'm going to tell you how small Raleigh is and how I have a theory that all the brown people know the brown people. People tell me it's just me that knows everybody. Larry's daughter signed me up for a personal trainer at my old gym. She's a runner as well. I've run into her at Diva myrtle and city of oaks in 2012.

They are making the race announcements. Then the race starts and we move up as the various corrals head out. Once our corral hits the timing mat I start my Garmin. We are off. Since I have not been running, I opt to walk. Garmin is running, I hit the play button on my playlist. I'm off and moving. Folks are passing me by as they are running down the street. I spy with my little eye the marathon has started on my left. As I head towards mile 1 I see my friend Natasha who is doing her first marathon and I yell her name. She waves back. I'm so excited for her, first full. I'm only 1/2 half crazy.

The pack is thinning out and it's just me and my personal stalker, Richmond police cruiser. The first 3 miles are the hardest and they ain't never lied. As I hit mile 3, I see a stadium and I realize this is where the expo was held the night before. I'm like holy Moly we are all the way over here. As we head to mile 4, I see folks coming up the road from where I'm headed and I see Sharon and Claudia. They ask me if I'm ok, I'm like yeah, I'm good. As I head out of the neighborhood I see a few cops on motorcycles and I realize the lead marathoners are headed my way. There they are 2 Kenyans flying down the street like it's nothing. I'm headed to mile 5, my personal escort has pulled closer and is in the left lane. A race volunteer heads towards me and tells me she needs me to get over in the left lane and head into the Park. Once I come out there is an aid station available with whatever I need to help me get to the finish.

I head into Bryant park. I see other half racers coming out. I get a few high fives from folks telling me to keep it up, you go this. In my mind, I'm thinking why am I out here and not back at the hotel chilling watching HBO. I'm in the park and I'm like good gracious where are we going, Maryland. This feels like the longest part of the course. I pass mile 6. Then I pass the 10K spot. The volunteer walks up to me and tells me to walk over near the timing mat so my time is recorded. I hear it beep and I think I've made it to 6.2 miles. Only 6.9 more to go. The sun is out and kicking my tail. I'm guzzling down water and I still have my PowerAde in my jacket which I sip on. I stop for a minute to get it together. My escort pulls up and ask me if I'm ok or if I need medic. I tell him I'm ok. I knew it was going to be a struggle and that's exactly what it was. I keep on walking and pass mile 7. I come to a turn and there is nothing to indicate what direction to go in. I turn around and ask the cop. He has no idea either. He drives up on the right and comes back and tells me he doesn't know where the course goes. He tells me to hop in with him. You think I didn't. We ride left and we see nothing with course directions. We come out the park out of a totally differ the entrance than we started. We turn onto a major road that is open so it's not part of the course and BAM we hit the course. He asks me what I want to do. I told him I'm finishing. I get out and head towards the course. The race volunteer from early heads to me. She tells me "I've been waiting for you" I tell her we lost the course. She apologizes and tells me they must have pulled up the course. I'm thinking to myself "no shit Sherlock". She directs me to the aid station and packs of runners are out now on the marathon course. I'm back on the course and I pass mile 8. At this point, we are going through neighborhoods, folks are partying all up and down the street. I see a house that is grilling. There's a beer station. Lady offers me a cup. I politely decline as I am that non-beer runner. I keep looking out for the infamous junk food station that's supposed to be at mile 9. I assumed I've found it as a volunteer comes over and tells me what they have and I tell her I'll take the gummy bears. I know the chewing will help me to keep moving, that's a tip I remember from Jeff Galloway training manual. My body is really starting to run down as I have just passed mile 10 and I stop in front of the medic aid station. One of the volunteers ask me if I'm ok. I tell her I need to sit for a minute. She offers me water and PowerAde, which I take. I'm feeling slightly better, I head back out. She tells me you only have 3 miles left. Only 3 miles, hmm. I tell myself I have a 5K left and that DNF is not an option. I keep thinking about the fleece blanket that finishers receive. That is my true motivation. One foot in front of the other. I hit mile 11, I decide to use my lifeline and call tall drink. I tell him to talk to me because I'm dead on energy. He is motivating me and suddenly I hear someone call my name and I turn around and it's Kat from Charlotte. We hug. She tells me she's so glad to see me. Kat says jo I'll see you at the finish I must knock out these 2 miles to get my medal. A little over 2 miles to go, I think I can I think I can. I see Virginia Union university. I'm thinking didn't my cousin Reggie go here and isn't this a HBCU and aren't they in CIAA. Tall drink is still on the life line and he says, "yeah jo they are". The course is FINALLY headed into downtown. I pass mile 11. I'm like 2.1 miles left to go. So, close but it feels so far. I'm walking through downtown. I pass through buildings that have VCU. I see 2 ladies pass me. I yell out "Priscilla is that you" she yells back "hey Johanna." The other lady says yes, it's Priscilla and she's headed to a PR. how cool is that. I pass mile 12. Guess who passes me as she heads to becoming a marathoner, Koren Atwater Townsend. She's looking great. Seeing Raleigh peeps heading to the finish line gives me extra energy. I'm getting real close. Folks are telling me you have 3 turns left and then it's a downhill finish. This totally random lady walks up to me. She asks me how I'm doing. I'm ok just ready to be done. She's a local race coach. I mention how I didn't properly train. She chastises me. I tell her but I've made it this far. She asks me if this is my first half. I tell her no it's my 5th. She replies really with the FACE. I'm pretty used to getting the face so smart-ass Johanna comes out. I tell her that I did shamrock back in March, 8K on Saturday and half on Sunday. Her face hit the floor. Don't judge a book by its cover. I may be 3 dollars and 6 dimes but these hips do get it in on the pavement. I didn't tell her that but I was thinking it. We get to the downhill finish. She tells me she came go any further. At this point I'm filled with every emotion known to man because I know I'm almost done. As I head down the hill, folks are cheering me on. I hear someone yell my name and its Angela Griffin from Raleigh. I see the finish line. I hear the announcer call my name. All I can think is thank God, this thing is over with. As I cross the finish line I see a familiar face waiting for me, my TRI sister Intisar is there. She gives me a hug and I hold on to her for dear life. I am a half marathon finisher again. I don't care that it took me over 6 hours. No, I do not.

Special shout outs go to my TIFL sister, Mary Hicks, Sharon Johnson, Claudia Gunter, Kat Collier and Intisar Hamidullah, my NCRC buddy Carolyn Quarterman and my tall drink Gregory Clanton. They all played a part in this journey. For that I say thank you.

Reindeer Romp

Charlotte, NC

December 12, 2015

I had heard about the Reindeer Romp on Facebook through the TIFL Alumni group page. I saw pictures of last year's race. I noticed the race participants received hooded sweatshirts. I love a hoodie. As fall drew near, I started to google the race and kept it on my calendar. I reached out to a friend who is from Charlotte to see if she was interested in doing the race as well. Then we could stay at her mom's house. Win-Win. Forward to a week before the race, my reindeer romp weekend partner informs me that she has another commitment and cannot make the race but she has planned with her mom for me to still stay with her for the race. SCORE.

The race was held on December 12, 2015 at the Harris YMCA in Charlotte. I drive down Friday afternoon. I make it to packet pickup at the Y just in time. As I turn into the parking lot, I spy with my little eye a car in front of me with a TIFL sticker. I think to myself well I bet that we are probably going to the same place. I indirectly follow them. I park and then I see the driver of the car is TIFL Charlotte past president Hillary Crabtree. I yell out her name and we head over to the Y. I pick up my packet and Melva's packet. Once I told Melva we were getting hooded sweatshirts she changed her mind in trying to sell her race bib. Good call.

I checked the weather before I left Raleigh and the forecast at 8am was 55 degrees. In my mind that's COLD. I opt to pack long sleeve running clothes. Since it's a Christmas theme race I pack my Star Wars ugly t-shirt. I'm up and at it Saturday morning. I have about a 30-minute drive from Mary Peed's house AKA Melva Peed's mom AKA my hostess with the for the weekend. I arrive at the Y about 7:26am. We are meeting at 7:30am for group picture. As I get all my gear out, I see a few TIFL sisters. I have now been designated the Raleigh exchange student. Isn't' that special? I will travel for a race. I'm starting to feel warm from the two layers I have on. I didn't bring anything else to put on. We head over to the race start. Our group is way too big for a groupie pic. We recruit someone to take a real group pic. Geri Hampton Jackson who has been designated the best Southeast groupie photographer gets one with her phone. After the picture, I go "pay the water bill". I see the crowd has dispersed. I just follow folks and end up at the start line. I'm walking this race as I have done all my races this year. I will return to running soon. I'm lining up with Angel and Tiffany and Alexia in the baby stroller. She has it the easiest and doesn't even know it.

At 8am, the race starts, we start on a slight incline. We make our way through neighborhood behind the Y. I'm moving along good with Angel and Tiffany. This course has some HILLS. The weather is started to warm up. It's foggy and humid. I'm sweating like a sinner in church in my too many layers of clothing. We pass mile 1 and we all are like it's just mile 1. I'm sipping on the water in my Camelback like it's the best thing since sliced bread. It really is because I am losing water from sweating like it's going out of style. The neighborhood is nice. We are admiring the Christmas decorations and the panther's decorations because this is Charlotte, home of the undefeated Carolina Panthers. We have just passed mile 2. I see another hill. I'm like come on. There's a cop out on the course who tells us "This is the last hill". Angel ask, "are you sure" He replies I have 2 weeks left on this job so I would not lie. Strangely enough he was right, that was the last hill. We make a few more turns after the hill. Angel tells me that we are making our way back to the Y because there is a traffic up and head. I'm so happy to see we are headed back to Sharon Road. The right lane is still blocked off for traffic. Our lovely personal stalkers, the race course pickup crew and the sweeper car tell us to get on the sidewalk because they are opening the road up. We get on the sidewalk and cross the intersection. We are about a block and some change from where I parked. We head to the finish; I tell Angel it's a shame my car is parked right there. She tells me nope we must make it to the finish line first. We run into Geri and Donella who are leaving. We run into another course monitor who directs on where to go to make it to the finish line. We meander through the parking lot and turn onto the sand and head to the finish line. The very helpful course monitor volunteers try to get us to run it into the finish line. I'm seriously looking at her like it's so not happening. I tell her I'm just happy that I made it. We all cross the finish line. My official time is 1:10:23. They hand us what looks like a medal but I am told it is a Christmas ornament. How cool is that? I wasn't even expecting any bling. I was SOLD on the hoodie. Another 5K is in the books. Back to back 5K's are done. 1 race left to complete for the year on December 19 in Virginia Beach, Surf-n-Santa 5 miler.

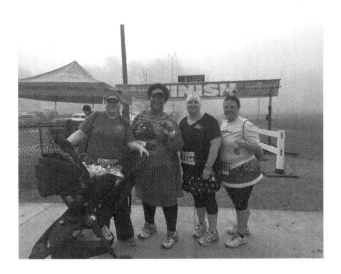

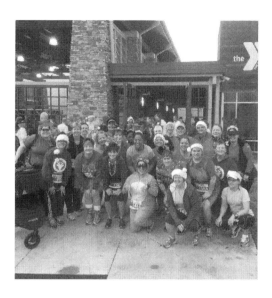

Surf N Santa 5 Miler

December 19, 2015

Virginia Beach, Virginia

Surf N Santa 5 Miler was my last race I was registered for 2015. It is organized by J&A racing. I have become a fan of this company since completing in Shamrock race back in March. They know how to do races and how to properly treat race finishers. I

I had heard about the race on Facebook through past participants. I truly enjoy themed races. I kept the race on my radar and kept an eye on the deadline for when the race entry would increase. I signed up for the race a few months ago, Then I reached out to my TIFL sister in Charlotte who is solely responsible for me becoming a fan of J&A racing, Angel Chappell Jonas. I checked to see if she was doing the race and she was. I went ahead and signed up. Now that I think about I may have signed up for this race back in the summer. I remember going to Huntersville packet pick up in Charlotte and running into Angel and we were discussing hotel arrangements. Yowzah I really did sign up early. That's the real way to save $ on race registration.

I booked the hotel through Hilton Honors because I am on a SERIOUS mission to earn enough points to stay at the Hilton Oceanfront resort in Virginia Beach during the summer. Hotel is booked. I was in Charlotte last weekend for Reindeer Romp. Angel and I were making final logistics for our trip. We decided since she was driving up from Charlotte. I would drive from Raleigh to Virginia Beach. It really made the most sense. We drove up to VA beach on Friday evening. Our first stop was packet pickup. We arrived at the convention center about an hour before race expo closed. We picked up our packets, hit the J&A store which I truly went into a conniption back in March buying everything that said 13.1 on it lol. This time I had much better control. I only purchased 1 shirt and 1-pint glass. Go me! We leave the expo and head over to our hotel. Siri is leading the way but everything looks completely different at night. Siri is a tad bit slow in telling us when to make the turns. We see the Hampton inn entrance AFTER we pass it. Thanks Siri. I end up turning into the exit instead of the entrance. No cop sees us so no ticket. We check into the hotel. Then go find some dinner.

The race is on Saturday at 4:30pm. This is my first evening race. I'm so used to having to get up at ZERO dark thirty for races. This is a nice change of pace. Get to sleep in on race day. Where they do that at?? We leisurely get up and thanks to Yelp we find a local breakfast spot. Carb loading at its best with the egg scramble. This decadent breakfast menu item is slowly putting me in a food coma. We make a stop at Walgreen's on the way back to the room. Then we are relaxing in the room to get mentally ready for the race. Did I mention the weather forecast at race time is 45 DEGREES? Baby it's cold outside. I'm a southern lady who LOVES the cold. I know go figure. I have brought lots of layering options. We decide to head over to the convention center, the START/FINISH of the race around 3. As we head over to the convention center, we see fellow races walking from their hotel to the convention center. Angel and I are both thinking "once they finish the race, they must WALK back to their room" No thank you. We make a pit stop at 7-11 so I can get a water for my camelback. I'm starting to learn my way around. We park in the lot. Then we make our way over to the convention center. I'm going to say ALL race participants are waiting inside before the race starts because it is a gaggle of folks in here. I make my way to the restroom and based on the line I am not the only one who had this idea. We wait around and do some people watching. People really go all out in terms of costumes. I even see a few Star Wars costumes, yeah!! Some folks are creative. The one that stands out to me is a guy dressed as Santa in a homemade sleigh with I'm assuming his girlfriend or wife dressed as a reindeer pulling his sleigh.

The announcer comes on over the PA system. "If you can hear my voice, you are in the wrong place. Head to the start line for the race" We leave the warmth of the convention center and head into the cold that is the start line. We are in corral

73

5. We line up with our corral. There is a wind whipping through which makes it feel about 10 degrees colder. I'm starting to rethink my life choices at this point. I'm here and there is 5 miles to get it in before I can call it quits. Race starts at 4:30pm. They move us out by corral. Our coral makes it to the start line about 4:41 minutes into the race. When you start a race with the crowd, you can easily get caught up with the hype of the crowd and start off to fast. I have had this happen to me a few times. About 5 minutes down the road, my body tells me to slow it up because this is not our pace. Angel and I are walking together. We are checking out the costumes while we people watch. We get passed by another Santa and reindeer. His sleigh has a sign that reads "Santa and his Ho Ho Ho's". Cute. We head down from the convention center and I'm not sure what the distance is but we are almost at the first turn onto Atlantic Avenue. I see the lead cars and cyclists turning to the convention center. We all scream out to the lead guy. Dude is flying towards the finish line. There is 1 other guy not too far behind him. We think wow he's already finishing and we are just starting. I think of the words Melva Peed told me "your race your pace". We head onto Atlantic Avenue. We hit mile 1. Right pass mile 1 is the first water stop and wouldn't you know it, it's right by our hotel. A part of me wants to make a beeline for the room. The way my bling obsession is set up I must cross the finish line. Also, the Max is parked at the convention center. We turn onto the boardwalk right behind Hampton Inn. As we turn onto the boardwalk, we are starting to lose daylight. They have holiday lights set up on the boardwalk. It is GORGEOUS. I've read on the race site that all runners must be off the boardwalk by 5:45pm. In my head, I'm thinking I can't really enjoy the lights because we must "fly like the wind bullseye" so we don't

get pulled off the course. We pass mile 2 on the boardwalk. I keep an eye out for The Oceanfront Inn because that's where we are staying for Shamrock. When I see it, I tell Angel "there it is". We booked it last night. Multi-tasking at its best. It's right at the finish line for shamrock. You have no idea how HUGE that is. This years' hotel was like a mile away. You may think that's not a lot. After you have just finished a half marathon another mile feels like 200 miles. We are coming up on another stop. I see all these folks dressed like gingerbread men. I don't see any cookies. Turns out they ran out of cookies. Story of my life for being the back of the pack. At this point, I am so ready to get off this … boardwalk. It feels like it's going on forever. I see the light show is ending. The last light display shows "Living the beach life" I figure I have time to snap a picture. Picture comes out good. We turn off the boardwalk and back onto Atlantic. We pass mile 3. We only have 2 more miles left to go. We head towards the last water stop right by the Hilton resort that I am obsessed with. The water stop is manned by what I am going to assume is college students because they are so HYPE angel and I are wondering what the heck did they have to drink and can we get some of it. We see a cop car head towards us and he tells us to get on the sidewalk. We get on the sidewalk. Literally 5 minutes later, one of the J&A race vehicles pulls up to us and tells us to get on the street because the course is still open. I tell Angel there must be a breakdown in communication because we have been told 2 different things. We get back on the road. We turn on 19th street to head back to the convention center. Angel can tell my breathing is getting really ragged. She gets my chews out my camelback. I was slipping and not taking my nutrition. I take a few stinger chews and guzzle some water and I get a 2nd life to make the last mileage to the finish. Angel tells me we are getting close because we can see the convention center. I tell her so close but so far. The course has going around the back of the convention center. This reminds of Reindeer Romp last weekend in Charlotte. As we make the last turn, 1 of the race volunteers walks up to us. She tells us she is going to walk us in. She tells us "I'm so glad you all didn't quit" I tell her of course not this is where the car is parked. She asks Angel if I have been joking like this through the entire race lol. We are coming to the final stretch; the finish line shoot is near and then we walk into the convention center and I see the finish line. I'm so excited that this adventure is coming to an end. It is so cool the finish line is inside the convention center. I hear the race announcer calling our names. There are a few folks hanging around cheering us on. Official finish time is 01:52. My last race for 2015 is

COMPLETE

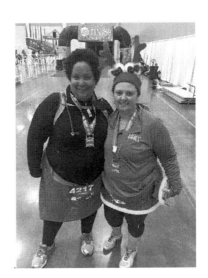

CHAPTER 7 - 2016

Lifetime Commitment Day 5K

January 1, 2016

Cary, NC

The best way to start off your new year than with doing a 5K. I along with a few sisters from my TRI Tribe decided to do the Commitment Day 5K at the Lifetime Fitness in Cary. Race started at 10am which is a good time since it's on New Year's Day and most folks have been taken part of adult beverages to ring in the new year. I personally only partook in 1 shooter early in the evening on New Year's Eve. I didn't even make to see the ball or the acorn drop as I was knocked out before midnight hit. I watched Frodo get on the boat with the elves in Lord of the rings: return of the king and then I was OUT.

I wasn't too sure what the parking situation was going to be like so I arrived at Lifetime around 9am. The gym was open for business as usual plus the participants of the race. This is great advertising for the club. It's what sucked me in about a year ago, when I joined the new club that opened in Raleigh. It's about 40ish degrees outside. I have on 2 top layers. I feel a wind hit me as I get out the car and decide I'm going to put on my hoodie. That was a good call.

I head into the gym to take care of some business AKA pre-race bathroom break. Good thing the race is at the gym so you have REAL restrooms. Oh yeah!! I pick up my fellow amigo Julie Reed's packet and put it in the car. By the time, I come back into the basketball court, more of the tribe shows up. I even see Mary Hicks is here. I haven't seen her since we did the Richmond half back in November. Good to see you Mary. Claudia and Sharon are picking up their packets. I see Barbara, Beth, Trish and Valerie. I even spy with my little eye Wendy Morris who I haven't seen since the finish line of Raleigh 70.3

As I tradition, we take a few pre-race pictures. Sharon is never without her handy dandy selfie stick. People are always amazed that I don't own one. I really can't say why I don't. Just haven't bought one. I am still accepting Christmas gifts.

We see people spilling out so we head outside as well. It's a little chilly outside. Yep good call on the hoodie. We head to the start line. Race announcer makes a few pre-race announcements. Then the race starts. Did I mention we start slightly uphill? The good thing about that is there will be a slight downhill finish, nothing like the Richmond finish. I head out with the tribe. I am walking like I normally do. I am really planning to step up my game this year and get back to run/walk intervals. It's just not happening at this EXACT moment. We turn left onto Regency. They have the lane closed off from traffic. Very nice. I heard a lady near me mention that's she doing the indoor TRI. I ask which one. She's says Cary. I tell her me 2. This is her first one. I wish her good luck. As I'm walking down Regency I see folks already on Swift Creek greenway. They are booking. Someone mentions there are probably folks already on Kildaire. I'm thinking to myself there is probably someone already headed to the finish. I have seen some of these super-fast runners finish 5K in like 15-16 minutes. I'm still heading towards mile 1. I have learned to accept that my race, my pace. I see these 2 ladies. I ask them if they did Jingle Bell

Run in Raleigh. The daughter tells me she thought it was me. Let me explain how we met, I walked with them during jingle bell run about a month ago. After we finish the race, the daughter tells me this was her mom's first race who is visiting from Brazil. She tells the mom that I'm the lady from jingle bell run in her native language which I'm going to assume is Portugal because it didn't sound like Spanish. Then again, I understand and speak semi-little Spanish. The daughter tells me the mother had asked her how much we had walked because the mother is about ready to be done. I so can relate. It's always like that for me at EVERY race. We hit mile 1 while on the greenway. Greenway is not as bad as I thought it would be. There are a lot of wet spots but nothing real torrential. I forgot my beats headphones at the house. I'm glad I did because without the distraction of music I really get to take in the scenery of nature on the greenway. It's pretty. I can tell I'm starting to get tired because my pace is slowing up and the group I was hanging with has left me. I'm cool with that. Just me, myself and I. I see a turn coming up and a course monitor volunteer. He tells me to watch it as I exit off the greenway because the path is kind of slick. I have a good sense of geography of Cary as I worked there for 16 years up until October 2015. I'm really trying to figure out where on Kildaire we are. I'm thinking we would pass the Wal-Mart shopping center. We turn left into a neighborhood and there is the water stop. They are still there and there is still water. Will wonders never cease? My race experience has taught me to bring my own source of hydration because I have come to water stops/aid stations and they have been OUT. I take the cup of water the volunteer is offering. It is like heaven in a cup. I am sweating like a hooker in church. I know I need the fluids. I keep walking past the water station. I pass mile marker 2. I think I only have 1.1 miles left to go. I can do this. Of course, I can, that is where my car is parked. I also have committed to doing the IRON KIWI challenge for January I need all mileage. The road through the neighborhood is slightly hilly. I take it 1 step at a time. I come up on the next turn, I see Cary PD there along with course monitor. They tell me I don't have that much to go. I thank them and keep on going. PMA (positive mental attitude) is on deck. I pass a few businesses and I see cars. I keep forgetting it a normal business day for some business even though it feels like a Saturday. I start to smell food and it is smelling good. I know I must be near the turn onto Tryon because Lucky 32 is coming up. I want to make a beeline in there but A. my money is in my car B. I will still have to walk to the car first. I bypass making the detour. I head towards Tryon. Course monitor tells me to stay on the sidewalk. I turn left onto Tryon and I'm getting excited because I know I only have 2 turns left. I turn left back on regency. They still have the lane closed. I see some people are leaving the race. This one car passes me and yells out "Black girls run dot com". That's probably the funniest thing I heard. I'm assuming they think I don't run because I was walking. I digress on the reason they felt the need to tell me about a running group that I am aware. I just nodded my head and kept walking. I'm heading towards the last turn. The volunteer is there who I passed at the beginning. She comes up to me and tells me "you are amazing, you are out here doing it and some folks haven't even gotten out of the bed yet" It's not about how fast or how slow you go. It's ALL about you making the decision to get out there and DO it. That's what I did. I crossed the finish line. As I was heading toward the finish line, I was very happy to see it was still up. I spy with my little eye one of my TRI sisters Wendy Morris is near the finish line. She comes and cheers me on. I tell her I'm so glad she was here and that the finish line was still up. My 1st race of 2016 is complete.

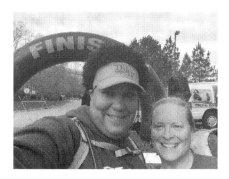

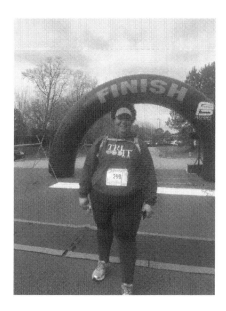

Shrimp & Grits 5K

January 16, 2016

North Charleston, South Carolina

I'm back in Charleston on MLK weekend. It must be Sharon Johnson birthday weekend. This year she's turned it up and there are 8 of us that have joined in on the fun. Claudia, Sharon and I learned after last year's race the 5K starts in north Charleston and not Charleston. We were staying in north Charleston so that made getting to the start line a few miles closer.

We arrive at north Charleston high school about 7:40am the start/finish of the 5K and the finish for the marathon/half-marathon. Race starts at 8am. As we walk to the start line we meet a TIFL charlotte sister Tulani. She thinks we are from the TIFL Charleston chapter. We respond no we're from Raleigh. RALEIGH in da house. My pre-race jitters are kicking in so I make a beeline to the portable restrooms. I run into Geri, Donella, Maryann and Stephanie from TIFL charlotte. TIFL is deep at this race. Yeah!! I find the rest of my peeps. Our Charlotte sisters find us and the southeastern selfie extraordinaire Geri takes our pre-race groupie. Sharon asks if she needs her selfie stick. I tell Sharon Geri is her own selfie stick. Say cheese.

We line up for the race. 8am we start off on the course for 3.1 miles. This is my 2nd time doing this race so I am familiar with the course. I haven't been running in like forever so I just keep walking at all my races. I got my music going on. RunKeeper and Garmin have started. I'm off on to knock out these miles. I pass mile 1 and I check my Garmin. I'm at 21:00/mile pace which is down from my normal 24:00/mile pace. That's what you call progress my friend. I slightly glance behind me to see if I'm the end and there are a few folks behind me. Woo Hoo I'm not the end. The water stops are fully stocked partly due to the marathon comes through part of the course. I pass mile 2 and I check the Garmin and I'm at 42:00 minutes. I'm so excited I've could keep up with the 21:00/mile pace. Since I've been moving like Jagger on the course I'm losing water left and right. I'm drinking from my camelback like it's the best thing since sliced bread. I know I'm less than a mile to go. I keep putting one foot in front of the other. I'm coming through the neighborhood. I know I have a few more turns and I'll be in the shopping center near the finish line. As I turn into the main strip of shops I see Claudia Mello's husband. He tells me I'm almost there. I notice he has on his medal so I know he's already finished. I make the last left turn. After I turn I spy with my little eye the mile 3 marker. I also spy some nice eye candy course monitors. :-)

I turn right past the mile marker. I see the finish line Chute up ahead. I make the last right turn and I see the finish line. I hear the race announcer. I hear the crowd cheering. So, I'm thinking they are cheering for me. Turns out the first male finisher of the half marathon is coming up right behind me. He finishes in 67 minutes, the same time I finished the 5K. I'm super Doppler excited I'm done but I'm also in awe that this guy just finished 13.1 miles in 67 minutes. Holy smokes batman. My 2nd 5K of 2016 is done. I grab my medal since the kids handing them out have forgotten they were supposed to be handing them out. I'm all about the bling. Did I mention as I was headed to the finish line, one of the volunteers who is a member of BGR Charleston walks up to me and invites me to join her BGR group? What is it about folks thinking I don't run when they see me walking? Who knows. I will eventually return to running. Especially since I am planning to qualify for half fanatics in 2 months.

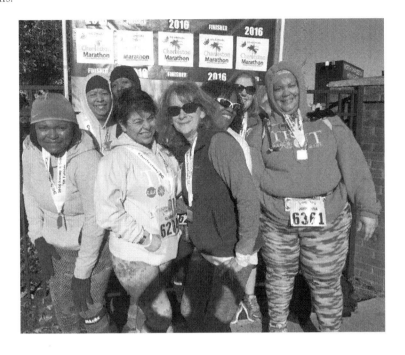

Run for the Roses 5K

February 14, 2016

Raleigh, NC

Today is February 14 AKA Valentine's Day. It also the 36th Annual Run for the Roses 5K held at the Dorothea Dix campus. When I parked at the race site, the temperature was 30 degrees. Baby it's cold outside. I had on several layers including a hoodie which I knew I was keeping on through the entire race. I even brought another hoodie to put on afterwards. What can I say once a Girl Scout Always a Girl Scout "Be Prepared"

Tall drink and his lady friend (we are not boys and girls, we are men and ladies) Donna Avery have signed up to do the race with me. I'm sitting in the car enjoying the heat. I see tall drink and Donna and he is motioning for me to get out the car. Pre-race jitters are kicking in and ALMOST don't want to get out the car. I get out. As I walk out to meet them, tall drink tells me I'm moving a little slow. I tell him it's pre-race jitters. He tells me there's nothing to be nervous about. I tell him whether it's race # 1 or #100 I will always get nervous before a race. It's part of the process.

We head into the gym, race headquarters. Tall drink and Donna must sign a race waiver since they just signed up yesterday. Tall drink is determined to get a race shirt. He confirms with NCRC President Rebecca Sitton on the shirt process. She tells him AGAIN they will pass them out at 3pm. I already know I will not be done in 60 minutes. I know someone who will because he wants a shirt. We hang out inside the gym and enjoy the warmth. Donna mentions to me "Jo there isn't a lot of brown faces

85

here" I tell her yeah, we come to races but we are always in small numbers. It is cold outside and you know how black folks feel about cold weather. I see a line starting to build at the ladies' restroom and I head on over and knock out this pre-race ritual.

Tall drink notices more folks are showing up. He says he's starting to get nervous. I tell him oh yeah you are ready for the race because that's a true sign. Rhonda Hampton makes an announcement that the race is starting in 10 minutes and all participants need to head to the start line. We head outside. As soon as I walk out the door, I am hit with a blast of cold air. I start to wonder about my life choices at this point. I'm already here so in the words of Fergie from The Black-Eyed Peas "Let's get IT started up in here" We head to the start line. I tell Donna I tend to hang in the back and let the fast folks line up in the front. I get the Garmin and RunKeeper set up. Race MC Brad Broyles announces the start of the race. We are off. Tall drink tells me he's going to walk with me through the race. I know he isn't because he has about a 12-minute pace. He sees folks running and he wants to take off with them. I tell him go ahead I know you want to run with them. I will see you all at the finish line. I don't move that fast. I'm not about to try today in this cold as ice weather. Off we go. We make the first right turn and I see Esther Dill on the corner volunteering as a course monitor. We head downhill and make another right turn and I see Louise Gardino. She tells me "Jo I'll see you one more time" As we head down the street, the lead cyclist is heading toward us with the front runners. Tall drink asks me "Are they already heading back" I'm like oh yeah, that's the front of the race. There's a brother in the front pack. What can I say I'm always checking for the other black folks when I'm at races? It's a reflex. We turn left and I see Paula O'Neal. Paula and I go way back to 2012 when she would always be my personal escort as the sweeper during races. She has since retired from Raleigh PD. we head uphill and this isn't even the HILL. It's waiting for us after mile 2. I am going uphill and I make a right and see another NCRC peep Jennifer Ennis. Right turn and around the back of the building and you get a nice view of the soccer field. Soccer folks are out today having a good time. I may need to find an interest in soccer because Beckham plays soccer and he's very easy on the eyes. I'm just saying. I will probably need to go across the pond and watch soccer. The big soccer tournament is coming up this year isn't it. No idea. I must ask google. Back to the race report. I hear Lisa Howell behind me and that means she is sweeping the race. We pass Jenn again. Then I see mile 1 marker. Woo hoo. I don't even check my Garmin to see what my time is. I'm just going to wait until the end to see what it is. Did I mention that my legs feel frozen? I thought they were just sluggish from yesterday's swim but oh no them jokes are cold. I keep pressing on. I see Paula again. 1 mile down, 2.1 to go. I can do this. Of course, I can. I'm self-analyzing what additional training I need to get in to get ready for tobacco road and shamrock. That's pretty much what I do during every race, I start to think about what I need to do better to improve my pace. crazy, right?? I take those thoughts out my head and I think about what Sharon Johnson says, "enjoy the journey". Since I've done this race before I know what I have left to do on the course. I turn left and head uphill. I come up on the water stop. I tell them no thanks to the water. I carry my own primarily because my experience is the water stops are out or have left the building. TRUE STORY. Pass the water stop. Lisa catches up with me. The couple she was sweeping has picked up their pace and passed me. They better do it. It's a husband and wife and they are getting it in. That's what I'm talking about. Tall drink

calls and checks on me. He's the best. He tells me once he finishes and gets his shirt,

he's going to come back and walk with me to the finish line. That's friendship right

there. We pass mile 2. Hallelujah. We are near the Boylan entrance and you can see a

nice view of the downtown Raleigh. As we pass the entrance, we turn left onto Tate.

Tate should be called the DEVIL because it a straight 90-degree hill from HELL. I

take it with short and steady steps. Slow and steady up the hill works well for me. I

don't stop for any breaks. That's called progress. we turn right and hit flat road.

YEAH!! We go around and then cross over Tate and I see Frank Hagg on the corner.

He tells me I have about 1000 meters left to go. I tell him I really believe you. I truly

know that there isn't much left to the finish line. We pass Carolyn Quarterman for a

2nd time. She walks with us since we are the end of the race. We talk about being at

Richmond together back in November. All cool people hang out at the same races.

Oh yeah!! I see an angel heading towards us, his name is Tall Drink. He comes to

walk with me to the finish line. He told me he got his shirt and Donna is in the car

warming up. He asks me how I'm doing. I tell him besides being cold I'm OK. We

make a right. We head down the street, pass the water stop. He tells me the finish line

is around the corner. I tell him this part of the race is the best because you know you

are almost done. We make the last turn. I see Esther, Louise and Rhonda. Tall drink

tells me "do you know everyone on the course?" I tell him well the race is being done

by North Carolina Roadrunners Club which I'm a member of. I know a few folks.

Lisa tells him yeah Jo is a veteran of these races. This is true. I see the finish line arch.

I also see the clock. I see 1 hour and 7 minutes. I can't remember what last year's' time was. I'm telling myself that I want to cross before it hits 1 hour and 10 minutes. I pick up my pace. Tall drink tells me "I see you picking up the pace" Lisa says "it's the race for the finish energy coming out" I cross the finish line in 1 hour and 8 minutes per Run Keeper. Lisa tells me "don't forget to get your rose" I pick up my rose. Another 5K is done!!!

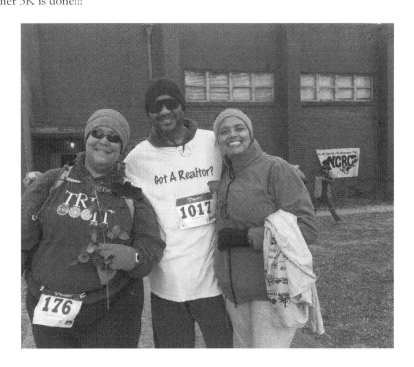

Tobacco Road Half Marathon

March 13, 2016

Cary, NC

I have had an interest in becoming a member of Half Fanatics. It's a group of folks who have done repeated half-marathons with a specific time. In my quest for Half Fanatics, I signed up for Shamrock half marathon on March 20, 2016 along with Tobacco Road half marathon on March 13, 2016. You can go ahead and call me CRAZY because I have accepted the truth that I truly am. Since I apparently missed the whole parking pass option when I registered for the race back in October, my parking option was the off-site parking at NetApp. Let me preface that I once upon a time attempted to become an employee at NetApp since all my former co-workers have gone to work there. I've heard it's an awesome place to work, up there on the list with SAS and MetLife. I digress. The parking instructions indicated that you needed to be at the off-site parking between 5am-6am to catch the shuttles to the race site. Since there was an expected 4000+ runners expected to be participating in the race, I opted to get there EARLY so I wouldn't run into any issue with catching a shuttle. With that in mind, I went to bed Saturday night about 9:30pm. Oh yeah that's how I do it on Saturday night the day before a half-marathon. Alarm clock was set for 4am. Yep I did not stutter 4am ladies and gentlemen. I popped up at 4am and slowly started my race preparations. Also, my brother from another mother AKA Tall Drink is doing his first half-marathon. I call him to check on him. I know he's up because he wakes with the chickens. He's wide awake. Dude sleeps like 2-3 hours, that's a nap in my book. We agree to meet at NetApp between 5-5:15am. I pull into the parking lot coming in through the back entrance apparently because there ain't a car in the lot. I notice there was a truck in front of me and he went around the corner. I ride around until I find civilization. BAM, I see green volunteer shirts. JACKPOT I have found the right parking area. I parked the Max and wait for tall drink to show up. This dude drives right past the place. "Big baby I see Cisco" I'm like you have gone too far. He finally turns around and finds NetApp. We gather our stuff and head to the shuttle pick up. I personally think the shuttles should just pick us up from NetApp that's Lazy Johanna talking. We walk to the corner of Louis Stephens and Kit Creek. Of course, the geek in me wants to google Louis Stephens later to find out why there is a street named after him. We cross over to the shuttles. Who do I see working with the police directing volunteers, Mike Waldvogel, a fellow NCRC member. We head to the shuttle and who do I spy with my little eye Paula O'Neal directing volunteers onto the shuttles. I know we are early because we are one the 1st shuttle. Shuttle is filling up quickly. We head to the race site. I ask tall drink how he is feeling, he's getting nervous. There are some extremely excited folks on the shuttle. Dudes shouting out to each other. An extremely chatty lady. Tall drink said she sure is talkative. I told him she's excited. As we head to the race site, I'm looking around at the route we take and I realize it's the same route I take to Mills Park where we perform our bike training sessions on Sunday with TIFL. It's a small world after all. Next thing I know we make a turn and we are here. That was quick. We unload and head to race HQ. I drop my gear bag. I inquire about t-shirt swap because female cut shirts are not meant for fluffy chicks. I'm told shirt exchanges will happen post-race. CHECK. My smedium shirt is in my gear bag. Once a girl scout, always a girl scout, be prepared. We have

91

about 2 hours before the race start. We find a bench and cop a squat. We meet a lady who has done the race for the last couple of years. She recognizes me from other races. She is wearing OBX half marathon shirt. I tell her I did that race in 2013. I run into my swim instructor Eric who is doing the marathon. I commend all folks who do marathons. I'm only ½ crazy. Per Ron Wahula, ½ crazy is still crazy. You got that right. I run into one of my TIFL sisters, Claudia Mello who is doing the marathon. We get a pre-race pic. Racing is all about the pics these days. Tall drink I run into my swim instructor Eric Kaufman who is doing the marathon. Claudia remembers him from the Lifetime-Cary running group. That's what I LOVE about this area. The running community is everywhere. They help you commemorate the experience. and I people watch some more. Since this is his first ½, he's taking it all in and he's checking out the eye candy. MEN SMH. The race announcer is bright eyed and bushy tailed and announces we should line up about 7:30am. I check in on my TIFL sister Kristie Pyle who drove up from Charlotte to do the race. That rascal is waiting in her car with the heat on. She tells me she will get out in time for the race line-up. She has 1 of those parking passes. She is parked like right at the start. IF I do this race again, I will drop $10 on the parking pass. You park like right at the race start/finish and can slide out through the back entrance. SCORE!!! I stretch my legs for a few minutes and walk around. I can tell by the crowds more folks are showing up. I run into one of my BTA sisters Candace Brown. She asks me if I'm doing the full or the half. I tell her I always crack up when I get asked that. I'm like I'm only ½ crazy but the fact you ask me is amazing. She tells me that means that she thinks I can do the full. Once upon a time ago about 8 years ago, I had a dream of doing a marathon. Then I watched the women's marathon during the 2008 summer Olympics. I saw Olympic trained athletes pass the … out. I decided that I no longer wanted to do a marathon.

As it gets closer to 7:30 we go and head to the line-up. Tall drink notices these green signs that folks are holding up. I explain to him that those are pace groups. Some runners run with pace groups to help them keep a certain time for the race. There is 1:30 (1 hour and 30 minute) half marathon pace group, we see 6:00 marathon pace group. I know there is a 7:00 limit on the marathon and then I see the pace leader and it's one of my NCRC buddies Marjorie. She has "attempted" to talk me into doing MCM (Marine Corps Marathon) a few times. "Jo come do MCM with us and get kicked off the bridge by the cops" First off MCM is a MARATHON and I ain't interested in doing no marathon.

As we wait for the start of the race, we run into Brittany and Ellen. I introduce them to tall drink. I tell him they just did Star Wars half in California. Ellen tells him Jo was so jealous of us. This is straight up TRUTH. Star Wars and Disney, that's what heaven looks like. I see Intisar and her sisters. They all have signs on marking her dad Matthew who is doing his 300th marathon. Completely AMAZING!!! Kristie finally makes it out her car and joins us. We are talking about the pace groups and she has now decided that she could totally do the marathon next year since you have 7 hours to complete. I tell her umm hmm I'll see you when you pass me while I'm doing the half.

The race DJ has some great music playing before the race starts. Final Countdown is playing. I crack up thinking about the Geico commercial. 8am is here and the race starts. Tall drink is called that for a reason and he can see the start of the race. He tells me they have taken off. We move towards the start. I tell him the race starts once we cross the start line. Once he crosses, he is gone like the wind. He tells me "big baby I got to set my pace" He moves way faster than I do and there was no way on God's green earth I was trying to keep up with him for 13.1 miles. He took off. I moved slow and steady out of the park which was slightly uphill. I break into a sweat already and we haven't even gotten started good. After I turn right out of the park I am really sweating and wishing I had brought a towel with me. I'm really wishing I would have brought my frog tog. Who would have thought about bringing a frog tog to a race in March which is technically still winter but today it feels like late spring? The roads are open and I notice I am the end of the race, my normal spot. There is no cop car following me like most races. I make the left onto Morrisville Parkway and I hit mile 1 and there is a water stop. I take some Gatorade. I make my way up and down Morrisville parkway. I'm like where is the turn onto the ATT. I see a cluster of people and cars and cops. I also see a lead cyclist heading towards me so that means the 1st finisher is done on the ATT and headed back to the finish. I see him, he is completely soaked in sweat. He is flying. I see the turn onto ATT. I turn left onto the ATT. After intense studying of the course map, drive-by of the road course on Friday and a bike ride on the ATT part of the course on Wednesday, I'm familiar on what the course is all about. I'm heading down ATT. I know there is another water stop coming up that my TIFL sister Meg Fanney is volunteering at. It shows up right at the White Oak trail head of ATT. My bladder is talking to me so I make a pit stop. I stop by and get some water and Gatorade. Wave to Meg and keep it moving. At this point I am feeling good. I don't even feel the heat at this point. I

94

believe my body temperature has dropped because my shirt is wet from the sweating. It's overcast and shady on the trail. I cross the trail crossing. Female cop is directing traffic. She sees me and tells me "you better do it" There is an abundance of encouragement at every race I do. I LOVE it. I keep walking down ATT. I pass the Galloway water stop. They have GU's and chews. I take 1 of each. I grab water and Gatorade. I see the water stop leader Cary Greening who is rocking a cool green Hulu skirt and matching hat. Folks are passing me on the opposite side heading back up ATT. I see a lot of my TIFL sisters, Meredith, Maureen, Beth, Miya, Jennifer. They are rolling on the trail. I am headed to another water stop. I see the sign and it's the BGR water stop. They have the Wobble playing. I can so tell my energy is -5000 because I don't even feel like attempting to dance to the song. DANGER DANGER!!!! I see Natasha Grimes passing out water. This is like déjà vu of 2 years ago, when she was going Race 13.1 Raleigh and I was working at the water stop and she was coming through. I remembered how she was looking. That's just about how I was looking. She came up to and asked me if I needed anything. I told her no and that this course was killing me. She told me "you know how we do, you got this". Did I mention my Bluetooth headphones had died about a mile or so back? I am no longer listening to my music. It's just the noise in my head which is starting to think we should just go ahead and call Uber to take us back to the park so we can call it a day. When you are racing, it is truly MIND OVER MATTER. Then sometimes it's your body trying to tell you. I am reminded of that scene in The Color Purple when the choir is seeing "God's trying to tell you something". I am headed towards the turn around and I am not doing good. I see Kristie on the opposite and she stops and comes over to me. She asks me if I'm alright. I break down that this course is kicking my ass. It's emotional at this point. She asks how I'm feeling and if I feel like I can keep going. She says, "Jo listen to your body, what is it telling you" my mind is telling me no but body is telling me yeah. I start to get it together and tell her I can keep going. She tells me to call her if I need anything and she will see me at the finish line.

I keep pushing along the trail. I see mile 6. I go through the tunnel which looks like something right out of a scary movie. It is cool in there but does not smell good. I am out of the tunnel and I keep thinking where in the heck is the turn around and I see a station set up in the distance but I see folks running past it. I'm thinking this must be the turn around. I see a sign on the ground that says half marathon turn around. As I cross the timing mat, the 2 dudes monitoring the timing equipment, tell me to turn around. Thank the Lord. I am officially at the ½ way point of the race. I head back up the trail. I pass through the tunnel. I pass the BGR water stop and get water and Gatorade. Carletta who I know by her FB name as Sea Jay offers me some potato chips. I'm thinking the salt will help me out. Negative will roger those suckers made me thirsty. I sip on my camel back and keep moving up the trail. I pass the Galloway water stop and get water and Gatorade. I ask for some chews. There is a sister passing out the chews. She tells me "your hair is so thick" I'm like oh yeah. She tells me "that's a blessing" I never really thought about it like that. Food for thought. I'm about 9 months into wearing my hair natural and it's like a mystery this thing called hair. I much on the chews and head up the trail. I'm really dragging. I keep stopping and leaning on the trees. One guy passes me and tells me you got the right pace, take your time and rest. He ain't never lied. I keep meandering my way on the trail. I hear a voice yell "Johanna" I know it's Eric, this dude is way too energized to be doing a marathon. He is running with Claudia. They ask if I'm ok. Claudia offers me some of her pickle juice. Thinking back a day later this offer, I should have taken her up on it. I tell them I'm ok. They keep rolling up the trail. I am telling myself I just need to make it to mile 10 water stop and then I am going to go take a potty break and sit down and get myself together. I am so happy to see the white oak trail crossing. The sister cop is still out there directing traffic, bless her heart. I see the sun is coming out. I'm like oh snap it's going to be blasting me once I get out the trail. I see a mirage in the distance. It's the water stop. EMS guy walks up to me and ask "if I'm Johanna? Folks have been worried about you. How are you doing" I tell him I'm doing ok just hot. He tells to go ahead and take a break at the aid station. I get water, Gatorade, ice. I take a squat on the bench by the tables. I see a female runner laying on the ground. EMS are around here. Next thing I know ambulance has showed up and they wheel her out on a stretcher. I tell one of the adult volunteers that it must be serious if they are taking her out. She tells that is the 2nd person she has seen be taken out on stretcher today. I hope she is ok. I grab the cup of ice they gave me. The wonderful volunteers have filled my camelback with ice and water. Hi Ho Hi Ho it's off to the finish line I go. 3.1 miles left AKA a 5K. I can do this. As I make my way to the trail crossing, I notice there are way less people out there. Guess the excitement is over and folks have hauled tail out of here.

I leave out the trail. I pass mile 11. I start feeling twinges in my legs. I shake it off. This was CLUE#1 that my body was telling me. I ignored it. I sip on water in my camel back that the lovely volunteers have filled with ice and water. Next thing I know both my legs cramp up on me and I am literally paralyzed and I hit the ground. I scream in agony because this is pain I have never felt before in my life. Folks show up to see what's going on. I have never experienced this in my life. I keep thinking well there goes my half-fanatic quest. One lady tells me she needs to be to sit up and drink the Gatorade she has in her bottle. I drink it. Another runner is massaging my left leg. I don't know who this dude is but he is an angel from God. Later I learn that he is runner with Galloway. It is helping my leg calm down. They are calling for help. A couple who was biking stopped to help. There are still good people in the world. I was truly down for the count. Medics show up and ask me what's going on. I tell them what happen. The seizing has stopped in my legs but I can tell they are still sore. 2 of the medics help me up. OMG that was hard to get up off the ground. They walk me over to their truck. I rest there for a while. Then it starts to rain cats and dogs. One of the medic says now it wants to rain. The rain feels good to me because I was hot and it's cooling me off. Just as quick as the rain starts it stops. I'm feeling much better. I get out and get into the SAG wagon. They drop me off down the road. I get out and start wobbling to finish out the course. I was so happy to see the entrance to the park I didn't know what to do. I hear this lady scream "you got this, you are almost there" I tell her she has the strongest lungs. This chick can holler like Marvin Gaye. I really am moving 1 step at a time because the legs are still sore and apparently, there is still something left in the tank. I keep moving and I see the finish line chute, I see Kristie on the side. She tells me "jo you are amazing" I keep moving and cross the finish line. I glance up at the clock and it's been over 6 hours since I started. Do I care that it took me 6 hours to finish, nope? I care that I finished and finished upright.

After I cross they give me my medal, thank you very much. This bling is huge. Me like ☺. I walk over to Kristie. I tell her I didn't think I was going to make it. I see Barbara Farrell another TIFL sister. She tells me she's been worried about me, she heard them talking about me in the medic tent. I see Intisar who saw me laying on the ground. She's so glad I'm doing ok.

As we are all talking there is applause from the crowd because the last Ansley Angel person is crossing the finish line. All their folks went out to bring them in. That's truly amazing. We get a group picture. I tell Kristie and Barbara that it is pure torture that after you cross the finish line, you must walk up a hill to get to the Race HQ. I see the RD and he gives me a hug and tells me that I have done something that 90% of people don't do and that's finish a race. Kristie is heading back to Charlotte. Barb is going to give me a ride back to my car that's at NetApp. First, I need to pick up my gear bag. Pick up my gear bag. I head over to the registration area and ask if they are still exchanging shirts. Ron Wahula is there and he tells me congratulations. Then he said, "you just finished a race and your priority is to exchange your shirt" I tell him "yep, brought my smedium race shirt in my gear bag". They swap my shirt out. Thank you very much. When I tell tall drink about it later, he laughs because he was the same way after run for the roses about getting a race shirt. I pick up the chocolate milk they are handing out. We stop by great harvest and get some bread. Barbara knows the lady. She insists we take a loaf of bread home. Well of course we did. Who turns down FREE bread. Not me. Barb asks if I want to get some pizza. I ask is it any good. She tells me I don't know any pizza that's not good after a race. I agree and respond it could be the worse pizza in the world but after a race it will taste like the best thing you have ever eaten. I walk up to the papa john's truck and the guy ask me if I want a slice, 2 slices or a box. I tell him if you are giving me the option of an entire pizza I will take it. Free whole pizza, free loaf of bread and 2 chocolate milks. I do believe I have hit the jackpot. With that ladies and gentlemen, Jo has the left tobacco road marathon and she MAY return next year.

Shamrock Weekend

March 18-20, 2016

Virginia Beach, Virginia

I never blogged about Shamrock weekend. It was such a whirlwind time after we got back from the race. Two days later, my mom and I were on a plane headed to visit my sister in Kuwait. Here is the short and sweet version. My mom signed up for the 8K at the race expo. We did the 8K together on Saturday along with a running buddy from Raleigh, Susan Hubbard. On Sunday, Angel and I trekked 12 blocks from our hotel to the race start in the pouring down rain. Mother nature was having another fight with #Bae as it was a Nor'easter. It was cold, raining and windy. About 3 miles in, my mother joins me on the race course. We finish the race together. Since she is not officially registered, she doesn't finish on the boardwalk. She goes down the bike path. Angel came and met me on the course to bring me in. She had already gone through the finish line chute. She still had on her race bib. I asked her if she could the finish swag and we give it to my mom since technically she did do the dolphin challenge even though she was not official. Angel and I both crossed the finish line. She got the finishers medal, beach towel, drawstring bag and hat. When my mom got back to the hotel room, I gave it to her. That made her day. The best memory from that weekend was my mom seeing me cross the finish line. This was the FIRST time she had been at a race that I was doing. She did the race with. I will remember that forever.

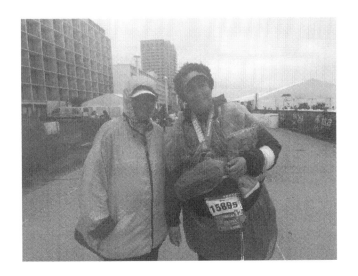

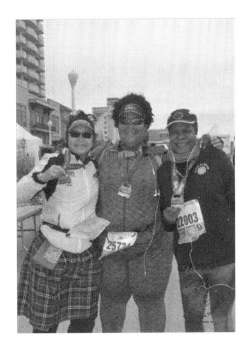

Rock N Roll Raleigh Inaugural 5K

Saturday, April 9, 2016

I am a semi-fan of the Rock N Roll race series. It's probably because I participated in the inaugural race in 2014. The weather went between 3 seasons and the course was from HELL. Myself and my partner in crime Sharon Mincey lost the course. I had so many ISSUES with that race. I was 1 and done. Since I've done a RnR race I am on their newsletter subscription. I received an email a couple of months that they were adding a 5K to the marathon/half marathon weekend and it also gave a glimpse of the bling. Once I saw the bling I was hooked. I had a made a deal with myself that if I ever did another RnR race that I would do a 5K. I was dragging myself in doing the registration. Then there some flash sale happening and they have 5K registrations for $25. Of course, I totally slipped and missed the $25. I did get in for $40 I was cool.

My mom has been hanging out with her 1st born since Shamrock weekend. I mentioned the race while we were in Virginia Beach. My mom was on board. My plan was to surprise her with race entry as birthday gift. My partner in crime Gregory Clanton told my mom that I should go and sign my mom up for the race. Totally not how I was planning it. I signed mom up for the race for the low low cost of $65. Mom is signed up for the race. We are out of the country for about 2 weeks. After we get back, we have about 3 days before race day.

We hit the race expo and pick up our packets and visit some of the vendors. Race is on Saturday morning with an 8am start time. I have discovered after reading race information that there is no parking on Dix campus. They are offering shuttle

103

service from downtown over to Dix. We opt to do the shuttle service. Shuttles are leaving from 6:15-7:15am. Mom and I leave the house about 6am. We park in the same parking lot that we parked for the expo. There is no parking attendant. SCORE, free parking. We sit in the car for a few minutes enjoying the heat from the car. My partner in crime, tall drink, arrives very shortly along with Donna and Shawnell. We all head over to the shuttles. The race organizers are running a tight ship. We line up and they load us into the shuttles. We arrive over at Dix in about 5 minutes. As we wait to board the shuttle, I spy with my little eye 2 of my TIFL sisters Tiffany and Ayuna. I call Tiffany congratulating them on arriving early. She tells me that I got her up at the crack of dawn and they are in formation lol. We unload the shuttle over at Dix. As we start to head to the start line, I see a black Cadillac pull up and I'm thinking that car looks familiar. It's 2 of my TIFL sisters Sharon and Claudia. I'm like you know you can't park here. She somehow has talked the volunteer into letting her park there.

It's about 7am. We have about 1 hour before the race starts. We go and cop a squat on a bench. We meet the other folks sitting on the concrete benches. Everyone is feeling the cold but I am not. After doing shamrock in a northeaster I can pretty much handle whatever weather mother nature wants to throw at me. At about 7:40am, the announcer tells us to start lining up by corrals. I am in corral 10. Ayuna is worried about the 1-hour finish time and moves up to an earlier corral. I tell her not to worry about the finish time. We are on a closed course at Dix. The race begins at 8am, they move us by corral 1-2 minutes at a time. About 8:10am, our corral is at the start line. I notice we have a slight uphill start. I pace myself and move slowly up the hill. As I am walking someone comes up behind me and taps me on my shoulder, it's my partner in crime tall drink AKA Gregory. He almost made me pee myself. That's what happens when you have your music too loud during a race, can't hear what's going on around you. I can tell that I've moving faster than I'm used to so I try to slow it down. I'm familiar with Dix campus as I have done a few races here. We make a left and head down and around and I can see the Raleigh skyline. I notice we don't go up Tate. We turn to go onto the green way. I notice I have my personal escort, cop car and cyclist. They leave me as I get on the green way. I hear the volunteer radio in "last runner is on the green way" Once I get on the green way I pick up a little speed and pass the group of folks in front of me, I tell them good morning and keep it moving. I'm surprised that I am passing people. It's normally the other way around. I pass another group. Greenway has a slight incline and I notice we are parallel to Western Boulevard. Then we exit off the green way and turn left back onto the road. We pass the soccer field where the shuttles dropped us. Mom ask me if we will pass the parking deck where we parked and I'm like no that's in downtown. I point out that we are passing by where the shuttles dropped off. I can see where the start line is. We turn right and we pass the water stop. Mom tells the volunteer she can't drink any water as she is trying not to have to make a beeline for the restroom. We head up another hill. I notice that we are on the same course as the women's distance festival from 2013. We turn right and I see a band playing and I pass mile marker 2. I see folks on the opposite side heading towards the finish. I see Ayuna. I hear Tiffany call my name. I high five Sharon. I'm thinking oh I got this because I have less than a mile to go. This part of Dix I have never been to before it goes through a little forest area.

It curves around and heads back. I pass the band again. The course starts to go downhill and I can see in the distance black tents and I know I am getting close to the finish line. A lady tells me "you are almost there" I tell her I truly believe I can see the finish line in the distance. I notice folks are lined up on the right. Then I realize this is the shuttle line. This line looks Black Friday line up at Best Buy. Folks have finished the race and RET to up out of here. I head towards the finish line. Another race is done. I stop my Garmin and check my finish time 1:08:19. Not bad, not bad at all. Especially for someone who just got off a plane from traveling from Kuwait 3 days ago, whatever you do, never ever give up!!!

Lifetime Fitness Indoor Triathlon
April 24, 2016
Raleigh, NC

Lifetime Fitness hosts an indoor triathlon twice a year. I enjoy participating in them. I signed up for the spring triathlon which was being held at the Raleigh location, which is my home club. Super excited. It takes me all a few minutes to get there. SCORE!! I wasn't sure if any of the TRI tribe was participating. Racing is always so much more fun when you do it with friends. I found out that one of my TRI sisters Barbara Farrell was in my same wave. Lo and behold I didn't even know her lovely daughter Heather was in our same wave. We are the 3 amigos for this race.

It is a lot easier packing for an indoor triathlon versus than an outdoor triathlon. There is no bike and no bucket. Since I know the gym towels are a little smedium, I brought my own. My TRI bag is packed to the brim with all my race day essentials. I make a pit stop at Panera for some pre-race fuel. I was all set to get my customary cinnamon crunch bagel with hazelnut cream cheese. When I pulled up to the drive-thru menu and saw the pictures for the egg soufflé I quickly changed my mind. They are life-changing delicious. I order the spinach and bacon egg soufflé and head on over to Lifetime.

As I pull into the parking lot, I spy with my little eye one of my TRI sisters Barbara, who for the record is a ROCKSTAR athlete and triathlete, walking towards the entrance. She asks me if I'm ready. I'm like oh yeah. After I check into the gym, I head over to the check-in table for the indoor tri. I receive my race bib and swim cap and race shirt. I opt for the red race shirt completing forgetting until after the race that I already own the red triathlete shirt. I later email the race coordinator about switching my shirt for the grey. I am still waiting on a reply to that request. It is a requirement to wear their swim cap which I think is going to be very interesting to see if ALL my hair will fit under it. Barb asks where the locker rooms are and I tell her they are around back like the Cary location. There is one set of stairs upstairs which is right by the women's locker room.

I head over to the locker room. When I go to the gym to swim I opt for a locker closer to the pool area. I head over to the 2nd to last row of lockers. I start getting my stuff out. I have seriously packet a lot of stuff. I must have thought I was going on an overnight trip. Suddenly, my stomach is doing its normal pre-race dance. I make a beeline to the restroom. I opt to go to the one by the pool to see the folks who are already on the swim portion. I see a TIFL athlete waiting for her wave to start. I can't tell you her name to save my life. I know she is one of our advanced swimmers. That's all I got lol.

I get ready for the swim. I stuff my hair into the tight swim cap. I head out to the pool area and wait for my wave to start. I talk to a few folks who are in the 9:40 wave. One lady I met told me this is her first triathlon. We talk about the swim portion. I think the swim is the easy part of a race. She thinks it's the hardest part. This is her first race so I can totally understand her thinking that. I ask if she plans on doing any more. She is thinking about doing one at the end of June in Philadelphia. Kudos to her.

Each wave has 10 participants. Our wave has 5 so we all get our own swim lane, SCORE. As soon as we get in the swim lane, we literally have about 15 seconds before the swim starts. Swim lead volunteer yells GO and I take off. Apparently, I went out way too fast because I for the life of me can't breathe when I go under the water. I'm really flaying in the pool like someone who does not know how to swim. Trust me I know how to swim but you couldn't tell today. I manage to squeak out 14x25 meters by the grace of God. Angela came up to me after I got out the pool and asked me what was wrong. She could see I was swimming like I was shook. I don't know what it is when I get to swim portion of a race but I get straight SHOOK. The exact same thing happened in Huntersville last fall. I got in the pool and couldn't feel the bottom because it was 6 feet and that FUCKED my head up for the first lap. After I got to the end of the lane, I calmed myself down and remembered oh yeah, I do know how to swim. I head to the locker room to change for bike. I'm dropping stuff left and right. Can you say frazzled? I'm changed into my cycling gear. Smart

Johanna packed gel seat cover for that tiny spin bike saddle and brought my cycling shoes. I have mastered the art of clipping in on a spin bike. I have not done as well on my road bike AKA Blue thunder. That's a work in progress. We head to the spin studio. Angela takes the elevator and I tell her I almost want to ride with you. Brittany, indoor tri coordinator, walks by me and tells me I'm so glad you didn't get on the elevator. I tell her I was really tempted but that would be sad to be taking the elevator while doing a race lol. Seriously I was really considering it. I chug up the billion stairs to the next level of the gym. Barbara and Heather tell me they are following me because they have no idea where they are going. We head into the cycle studio and the spin volunteers tell us to find our bike based on our race number and that we are 3 minutes behind, like I care I have lost 3 minutes on the spin "death trap" bike. I get my bike adjusted. I put on my gel cover. I get my water and sports beans out. Hydration and nutrition are very important. I hop on the bike and attempt to clip in. Right clip is in, let's get the left clip in. Volunteer turns the computer on and off I go. It's been a few months since spin class. I got to tell you it is nowhere as bad as it was about 15 months ago, when I was on the spin bike for the very first time and I thought I was going to DIE. Apparently, I didn't because I'm still alive. I personally don't think they have the air on here on purpose because I am sweating like a sinner in church (princess and the frog reference). I'm about 15 minutes in and I have knocked out 3 miles. I'm thinking to myself my goal is to finish with 6 miles. Just keep pedaling. Spin bike is not that bad today. Could be the extra padding I brought with me to ease the pain. I'm coming up on 6 miles. I hit 6-mile mark. We still have a few more minutes left. I'm thinking let's go for 7 miles. I go for 7 miles.

Spin instructor tells us we have a minute left. I'm really trying to make 7.5 miles since I was born in 1975. She calls for us to stop and I look down and I am at 7.4 miles. I'll take it. We have 5 minutes to head over to the treadmills for the run. In the 2 years, I have been doing triathlons I have never run during the run portion. What can I say my body is so happy to be off the bike we just get on the run course and just move one foot in front of the other but not as fast as most folks. I head to the treadmill. I get my phone and headphones out and get my playlist going. 20 minutes on the treadmill. My normal pace is between 21-22 minutes. I already know that it will be a Sunday morning miracle if I hit 1-mile mark today. I start the pace at 2.8 to warm up the legs. After a minute, I move it up to about 3.0. Oh yeah, we are warmed up now. I get a little adventurous and move it up to 3.4. The drill sergeant AKA tall drink told me that 3.4 should be my goal on the treadmill to get to the pace that I want on race day. I hung out at 3.4 for a few minutes. Once my heart started beating and the sweat was dripping into my eyes that was my sign to cool my pace down and I slowed it down to 2.8 for a few minutes. We were not on the treadmills in the gym that I am familiar with that tell you what your pace is so I had no idea what mine was at. I toggled back and forth between 3.0 and 3.4. I noticed my mileage was getting close to a mile. I also noticed I was running short on time. The run volunteer was counting down the stop clock and when we were done, I saw my mileage was 0.95 miles. I was very close to a mile and that is amazing. I have completed my 2nd triathlon for 2016.

Diva North Myrtle Beach 5K

May 1, 2016

North Myrtle Beach, South Carolina

I have felt that Myrtle Beach was cursed for me in terms of races. Let me provide my evidence to support this theory. Exhibit A, 2013 I participated in the Diva half marathon and because my pace was below their required 16:00/pace I was picked up by the SAG (snatch and grab) van. Exhibit B, 2014 I participated in the Myrtle Beach half marathon and I started having a mild panic attack at mile 8 and was put on the medical van. So, do you see why I have felt MB was cursed. A very good friend of mine Melanie Shaw, who has been motivated to do races wanted to do the Diva race. I told her the only race I will do at Diva is the 5K. I know I am not fast enough to keep up with their 16:00 minute pace. The both of us signed up to do the 5K. After mom and I got back from Kuwait, she signed up for the race as well. My mom has completely drunk the Kool-Aid.

My mom and uncle met me in Myrtle on Saturday the day before the race. We met up at the race expo. I had been there for a minute by the time they arrived. My mom picked up her packet and checked out the vendors. She got to meet a few more of my peeps, Theresa Hunter, one of my TRI sisters. She met Laura and Sevanne and their mom Rita, who came down from Raleigh for the race.

I booked my hotel through a recommendation from my friend Laura. I am so glad that I did because it was across the street from the finish. It was like a block from the start. DOUBLE SCORE!!

The 5K started at 7am and the half started at 7:10am. Since my hotel was so close. I was up at 6am. I headed out to the start around 6:35am. I kept calling my mom to make sure she was headed to the race as her hotel was about 19 miles away. As I head to the start line I run into Melanie. We head to the start line. It's getting close to 7am. The announcer is starting to do the countdown, I call mom again to see where is. I tell her the race is about to start. She didn't realize it was starting at 7am. Race is off. My mom isn't here. I head out with the race but a part of me is not into it because my mom hasn't made it yet. I start the Garmin and RunKeeper. I start to set my pace. The course is looking very familiar since I have been on it before. The first mile turns onto main street behind the finish line. We go right past the golden griddle pancake house. FYI this is the BEST breakfast spot at the beach. I'm thinking what I wouldn't do for a hot stack with eggs and bacon right about now. Food later, race first. I pass mile 1 and I decide to check the Garmin, my pace is about 21 ish minutes. This is not bad. I was trying to get to a 20:00/pace but I haven't been walking due to my plantar fasciitis. I keep on moving. I pass the water stop. There are some ladies who run to the water stop screaming out WATER. I laugh to myself because that is exactly why I always bring my own water. I do take the water that is being offered to me by one of the volunteers. I pass the water stop and keep moving. It's only in the 70s but the humidity is ON. I have been sweating like a sinner in church since about ¼ mile in. I'm thinking I should have grabbed a hand towel from the hotel to wipe the sweat. Oh well. You always think about what you should have done after the fact. That's the way it goes. My phone rings and its mom calling. She has made it to the race and is on the course. She has just passed mile 1. I tell her I just

112

passed the water stop and I will wait for her. I am so happy that she has made it. I see

her coming by way and I take my phone out to snap some pictures. She is so happy to

see me. We start walking together. She tells me that she was getting down that she

might miss the race. She parked her car somewhere. I tell her we will find it after we

finish. Mom thought it would be cold for the race because it was so cold last night

with the wind. I ask her it's warm out isn't it. She just laughs. We make a right turn

and head to the turnaround. After we pass the turnaround, there is a group playing

music and a couple dancing. I tell mom this is shag country. She's like what's shag. I

tell her it's a form of dancing and it looks like Chicago stepping. The group has some

great music playing. Mom is dancing while she is walking. She is loving' it. As we

walk, we look to the right and see folks on the last stretch to the finish line. Then I

see a guy on a bike past us. I'm wondering if this is the lead cyclist. He turns into a

driveway. Then a cop car rides past us and tells us the first half marathoner is coming

through. This chick FLIES by us. She is moving so gracefully that it doesn't even

seem like she is running. I'm always amazed at the fast runners because they look like

they are flying. They make it look so smooth. I told mom I knew the first finishers

would be catching up with us. Then I remember they have more distance to go than

we do. Then I'm wondering if we have missed our turn. Right after I say that, our

turn is coming up. I tell mom we not trying to miss our turn and do another extra 10

miles. No thank you. We make the 5K turn and then make the turn onto ocean drive.

We are truly in the home stretch. Mom tells me she thinks this is where she parked

her car because it was near a place named Alta Vista. We come upon the tiara and boa

station. Little girls are passing them out. They are too cute. I tell you I'm not all happy about that feather boa. My neck is ringing with sweat and the boa sucks it all up and it's making me hotter. We are coming into the home stretch. We make the right turn onto main street. People are lined up on the sides cheering us on along with the other folks heading to the finish line. We cross the finish line. I look up at the clock and it reads 1 hour and 20 minutes. I don't even care how long it took us to finish. I am just happy to have finished another race with my mom. That's a memory I will cherish forever. After we cross the finish line, they are handing out water. I'm like where is the bling. We turn and there is the bling. I almost forgot. There are shirtless firemen handing out the medals. Mom sees them and yells "Johanna pull out your camera" She tickled pink about this. I get a picture with her and the firemen. They put my medal on. I take a picture with them as well. This is how you finish a race. Bling and eye candy, YES!!

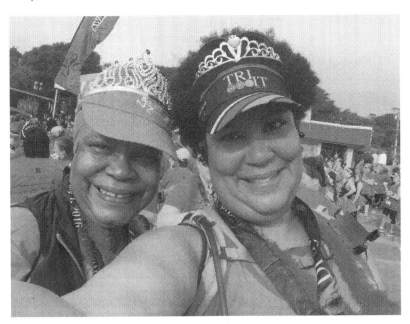

Smile Train Triathlon

June 26, 2016

Wake Forest, NC

This race seriously had me contemplating giving up on doing triathlons. I was at that place in my head for a good portion on the bike course. I will get into that during bike course recap. Before I get started I want to recognize folks who without their help and support today, I would probably still be out there riding aimlessly on the back roads on Wake Forest. Wake county sheriffs who were my personal escorts from about mile 7 up until I cross over heritage lake road back to the bike dismount line. FS series SAG wagon who was behind me probably 3 quarters of the bike course and I didn't even realize until about the turnaround at mile 6. My TIFL tribe who is always there for love, support and motivation. I especially want to thank Heather Leigh who walked with me on the run course. She probably saved my life and didn't even know it. Alexis who rode her bike on the run course to bring me some water and to see where we were. Even though she talked junk to me because I declined the water because I always have my camelback on me with water. Chris McDougall who took my bike and TIFL bag and walked them to the car for me. Post-race I was pretty much dead inside.

Transition opened at 6:30am. I woke up 2 times before my 5:15am alarm. That's how it goes on race day, your body is paranoid that you are going to oversleep so you keep popping up checking the time. When the alarm went off I was ready to get up. I'm up getting ready and after eating my bowl of cereal I'm like well I guess I will get on out here and it's about 5:55am. I'm about 15 minutes from Heritage where the race is being held. I get there in no time. Waze takes me the back way on Louisburg to Forestville road. As I get closer to the swim club, I notice folks are parked on the sides of the road. I'm thinking this is interesting race parking. I barely remember something about parking in a lot about ½ mile from the race site and ride your bike. That got me messed up thinking I'm riding my bike before the race start. No thanks. I pull into a spot on the side of the road. Benefit #1 of showing up early you get a close parking spot. I unload all my stuff. This is my first tri without using a bucket. Look who has grown up. I got my bike, tri bag and camel back. I cross the street and walk up to the race site. I find my row in transition. I'm 302 and the row starts with 301. Guess who mounted her bike on the beginning of the rack. Benefit #2 of being early, get the good spot on the bike rack. I spotted Karen and Ron Young when I parked. They are setting up their transition area. I find my towel and start pulling my gear out. I grab my race belt and head over to registration to get marked. It's about 2 blocks around the corner. I sure am lazy for a triathlete. What can I say I am probably the laziest triathlete you will ever meet? I get body marked. Volunteer asks me my age and I had to think about that because in triathlons your age is what you will be in the year. My age is 41, holy smokes batman when did I leave 40. Thank goodness, I still have less than 2 months to enjoy 40 lol. I head back to transition and I see a few more of the tribe show up. Cynthia rolls in after picking up her race packet. Alexis rolls in like a boss with her fly shades on. I see Teresa coming in. Claudia comes in. Kathy/Patty relay team comes in. Mary and John come in. I spy with my little eye Sharon Johnson from afar talking to a volunteer. We get together for a pre-race photo. Karen tried to NOT be in the photo. That's so not happening. I tell her when a person doesn't want to be in the photo, they must be dragged into the photo and that's exactly what happened.

I'm wondering about the restroom situation. Another racer tells me the bathrooms are locked at the pool. I was really hoping to use a real restroom. Like the Geico commercial, "not in my house". Heritage ain't playing it. You scrubs go use the porta potty. They probably didn't say that but I bet it was something real close to it. ROFLMAO. I make the pre-race potty run. I start to re-think my race attire. I don't own a real tri suit. It's hard out here for a fluffy triathlete. I opt to wear my swimsuit that I train in for the swim portion. I brought my cycling shorts to put over the swimsuit for the bike portion. I brought my run shorts for the run or as I like to call it recovery let's just put 1 foot in front of the other and move portion. It's a bit of a process when you must use the bathroom with a 1-piece swimsuit on. I head back to transition. I'm thinking whoever set this up wanted us to really get some walking in if you had to go because you must go back up a hill to get back to transition. I told you I was lazy right. Yeah you are starting to believe me aren't you.

Pre-race meeting starts at 7:45am. We head over to the pool. The microphone system they have is apparently owned by Chick-Fil-A because it is not open on Sunday. Race director is attempting to talk to us. I can barely make out what she is saying. I realize the swim is starting because the first group is lining up in the pool. The pool looks so good. I just want to stay in it all day. Since my race number is 302 I have some time before I start. We hang around and watch the first swimmers. They move so gracefully and fast in the water. Before you know the 1st swimmer is out, some teeny bopper. No, I am not hating. It was a teenager who came out first. I

117

see the first female come out. I see the first chip come out. Chip = a person of color. This comes from my fellow TIFL & BTA sister Dawn Davis-Calhoun. I'm always on the lookout for the chips at the race. Sharon finds some seats in the shade. Yes, I will come take a seat in the shade. Sharon knows me and heat do not get along well. More on that combination later. This waiting process helps my pre-race jitters to calm down. We see Alexis in the pool and Kathy. I walk over to see her swim. I've noticed the 200's are in the pool. I head on over and get in the waiting area. I was expecting the water to be cold. It felt so good. I told Cynthia why can't we just stay in the pool the entire race. Unfortunately, this is not a pool only event ☺ We line up. She's 300 and I'm 302. 301 must have gotten smart and stayed in the bed, smart person. As we are in the water, a couple behind me ask me if this is my first race. I'm like no this is my 5th tri but first time doing this one. They are amazed but they don't give me the LOOK. You know the one I'm talking about. Then they tell me they are runners and they just decided to sign up. They were not prepared as they don't even goggles. Did I mention they weren't wearing swim caps? Bless their little hearts.

The swim portion is beginning. Cynthia goes first. Then I line up and the timer tells me go. I push off and enjoy floating and then move into freestyle. I remember what my swim coach told me long and smooth strokes. That's what I do. I was having breathing issues. It's one of my weak areas in swimming. I didn't have any form of a panic attack like I did back in April at the indoor tri. I didn't even count how many lanes I had left. Just like Dory said, "just keep swimming just keep swimming." On a SN: if you have not seen it yet, do yourself a favor and go see

Finding Dory. I will go with you because I enjoyed it just that much. Baby Dory is just 2 cute for words. Back to the race. I'm about 25 meters from being done, I hear Candace tell me "Jo you only have 25 meters left to the finish now show me some form you're on video". I'm almost done, woo hoo!! Sweet baby Jesus let's knock this thing out. I swim to the end and I spot the ladder and head to. Why am I having issues with using my legs to lift myself out the water. Minor technical issue. I get out the pool. The tribe spectators are there "jo you're done next up is the bike" I head to transition and find my spot. I attempt to put on dry cycling shorts over wet swimsuit. It was comical if I do say so myself. Bike helmet on. Socks and shoes on. I have clips but opted to not try clipping in today as I am still learning that process. Camelback on, nutrition in camelback. This is the one time I opted to NOT bring my phone with me. That was a rookie move which I contemplated on later. I head out with my bike. Volunteer tells me to watch out for the curb. I head to the mount line. I am having some serious technical issues I have one bike glove, for the life of me I cannot get the 2nd one on. I drop it not once but twice and the very kind volunteer gets it for me. He asks if I have ridden this course before. I tell him I tried to drive it yesterday but got turned around. He tells me there are some hills and speed bumps in the neighborhood so be aware. I get on my bike cross the street and can you believe I cannot pedal. My bike is in torture gear. As I think back on this now, I should have taken my bike for a spin around the neighborhood after I picked it up Friday from Performance. Another rookie move. I am full of them today. You would have thought this was my first tri and not my fifth one. The beginning of the course goes up a slight hill and I am in the wrong gear and for the life of me I can't get out of it. I am working up this hill and it's

119

a struggle. There's a picture of me on Facebook at this exact moment and my facial expression tells it all. I make it up the hill, I get my gears straight and I'm off. Why are my legs already tired? Jesus take the wheel because this is going to be a struggle for real. I'm rolling through Heritage. There are hills in this neighborhood and I am reminded of Preston with Le tour de Femme bike ride in October. I struggle up the hills, if you know me this is serious progress. I would normally hop off the bike and walk up. Not today I am trying to put the spin classes to use. I make it through the neighborhood. Turn right onto Chalks. Here comes another hill. I see Alexis heading back telling me to take that hill down. I don't know about you but I don't get real encouraged when I'm on the bike course and other folks are yelling stuff at me even if it is encouraging. It could be that my PMA (positive mental attitude) was at -5000. What can I say I was not a happy person on the bike course? Everyone who saw me felt it. I'm making my way on Chalks and I'm thinking to myself isn't this the road my ex-fiancé's mom lives on. I pass a turn for a radio station and the next turn is for her house. I see a sign that reads organic eggs, cage free. I'm like I don't think she was into farming but who knows. I'm like I know exactly where I am and this is about to get real hilly because I can recall riding on this road. It does and I push on through the hills. Whoever told me the bike course was flat was a LIAR and I'm giving you serious side eye right now. I get to the intersection and turn left. I pass Jones Dairy road the street I was on yesterday after I got turned around trying to find the bike course. You really get to see a lot of Wake County when you are out here on these lonely roads. I kept singing in my head "All by myself, don't wanna be all by myself". I come to the next turn and make a right. I'm getting real close to the turnaround.

120

Thanks goodness. The hoo ha is not happy with me. Neither am I. It's hot out here. I'm ready to be done. I really want to just go home and lay on my recliner. I start to accept the fact that I will take a DNF on this race because I am just not feeling this race today. In my head, I, had accepted the fact that this triathlon was going to become a duathlon if I can just survive the rest of this bike course. When I feel a need for a break from the saddle, I hop off the bike and walk. I hear a car approaching. It's the SAG wagon, they ask me if I'm ok. I'm like just took a break off the bike. I get back on and I head towards the next intersection. I turn left. Volunteer tells me it's not that much farther to the turnaround. I pass mile 6. This is a setup. The turnaround is past mile 6. I see the lonely course monitor directing me to turnaround. I hop off the bike and get some nutrition out my camelback and then get back on. 6 miles done and 6 miles to go. I think I can I think I can. I head back and I turn right at the intersection. Thank the volunteer and wake county sheriff. I keep on pushing. I pass mile 7. I get off and walk some. SAG wagon pulls up and ask if I'm ok. I tell them I am and they tell me they are back here if I need anything. When you are the end of the bike course, you get your own personal escort the SAG wagon. I turn left at the next turn. I notice the cops that were at the Chalks intersection are headed towards me. I'm thinking is there no one at the turn. White dodge charger pulls up in front of me with his blinkers. It's a Raleigh PD. He leads me and SAG wagon follows. Oh yeah, I have my own entourage on the bike course. How I wish someone could have taken a picture. We all turn right onto Chalks. There is some downhill. The charger sees me lower my head because I am embracing the downhill and rolling about 19 MPH. I struggle uphill but downhill in the words of Ludacris "move get out

121

the way." The charger picks up speed so I don't run into the back of him. I head to the very last turn, halleluiah. Make the left and I'm back in the lovely heritage neighborhood with their wonderful hills and speed bumps. A complete random stranger rides up to me and starts talking to me. Tells me he lives in the neighborhood but he's not doing the race. We come to a hill, he gives me a push and tells me he and his wife bike all the time. He does the same thing for her to help her up the hill. Thank you, random stranger, because you my brother has become my HERO today. There is another hill and speed bump. I make it up it. We pass the golf club. We head back to the race site. I have never been so happy in my life. When I passed mile 11 I got real emotional because very honestly, I didn't think I was going to make it. I cross over heritage lake and dismount. Barbara stone-newton is there rooting me on. 1 of the FS series guys comes over to me congratulating me on finishing the bike course. Then he tells me has some bad news, they are opening the roads on the run course and unfortunately, I'm going to be able to do the run. I tell him you say that like it's a bad thing. In my head, I was already out after the bike course. I head to transition, drop my bike. I see a few of the tribe and tell me that what they said. Then I go ask another FS official if I go do the run course on my own will I still get the medal. 1 more FS official and race director later I am given the green light. I go put on my visor and race belt, grab my PowerAde, suck it up buttercup because you are about to do this. I head out on the run course. I pass the tribe who is chilling in the shade. Yes, that is hate you have detected. I wanted to be chilling in the shade as well. Oh well that's the life of a turtle. I'm walking on the course. I hear some shoes flopping behind me. You know what it is. It's the sound of an angel named Heather Leigh who is coming to walk with me. I'm so glad to have the company. We walk the course together. We admire the gorgeous homes in the neighborhood. The SAG wagon passes us to check on us a few times and to make sure we're still on the course. Heather tells me she came with me because she heard someone was giving out beer and doughnuts on the course. We found doughnut pieces on the ground but we never found the house. The mile markers have been removed so I have no idea how far we've gone. I see another hill and I'm ready to turn back. We head back. I am so over these HILLS. I thought the bike course was disrespectful. I knew the run course was hilly with no shade. The run course was what I had been worried about for weeks. I kept drinking from camelback and alternating with the PowerAde. We turn back onto heritage lake. We see Alexis riding towards us on her bike. She tells us she brought me some water but I have my camelback. She tells us she will ride back to tell the rest of the tribe I'm almost done. We pass by the parking lot that was reserved for race parking. I tell heather ain't no way I was parking there and then climbing the hill to the race site. We climb the hill and we make it to the 2nd to last turn. Volunteer tells us we have 1 more turn and we're done. The last turn has a slight incline to it. We push on up this hill. Angela is still on the corner. I tell Heather I guess the rest of the tribe rolled out. As we get closer, the course monitor yells out "jo you go this, you're almost done" I tell her I am done. She replies no once you make it across the finish line then you will be well done. I laugh. I make that left and the McDougal family is there waiting. Kimberly is at the finish line with her phone. The timing mat is still up. The clock is still up. They haven't shut down yet. I cross the finish line. I am officially DONE DONE.

24 Hours of Booty

July 29-30, 2016

Charlotte, NC

24 hours of booty is a 24-hour cycling event that benefits cancer organizations. I was a booty virgin, I borrowed that phrase from one of my TIFL Charlotte sisters, last year. I really enjoyed it and decided to come back for round 2. When you sign up for 24 HOB you commit to raise $400 to ride. Back when I was employed, fundraising I thought was easy. I would strategically solicit my fellow co-workers on payday Fridays. The company has a matching gift program as well so that would double the donation. As most folks know I became unemployed October 2015. Now fundraising is like pulling teeth. I started off with an email chain to a few people. I also used social media. With a lot, more soliciting friends and family I finally met my goal of 2 days before the deadline. It was down to the wire.

I left Raleigh Friday around lunchtime and headed southbound on 85. After running into standstill traffic, a couple of times and finally stopping for lunch, I made it to Booty Ville around 4. Booty Ville is where riders camp out over the course of the next 24 hours. They may have had this last year and I just wasn't aware of it. They have a gear drop area. I pull into the drop off area. There are volunteers to help you unload. I tell them I need to give them a tip. The 2 teenagers laugh at me and tell me I'm doing the real work I'm riding. The TIFL tent is easy to spot, it's bright pink. I set my chair up and take a break and drink some ice-cold water. A sister came ready this year. Packed the big cooler with all kinds of hydrating beverages. I started off with 2 bags of ice when I left Raleigh. By the time, I get to charlotte I'm down to ¼ of a bag of ice still intact. The heat is on!! I see my buddy Kristina Blake. She drove down from Pennsylvania with her cousin. That is true commitment right there. Right after I pull in, our booty coordinator Laurie Certo pulls in right in front making another drop off stuff. After I cool off, I go park my car. Then head back over to my home for the next day.

The ride officially starts at 7pm. I opt to go shower before heading out. Did I mention there is a full shower facility in the Levine center that is at our disposal? SWEET!! Guess who headed to the locker room without her towel, this chick. I improvised. I have learned from last year to not go out at the beginning because it is a mosh pit of riders. Angela Stevenson and I decide to go out about 7:20. We head out. My personal goal is 25 miles. My plan of attack was to do 3 loops at a time. That would be 9 miles. I'm on the booty loop. I remember that it starts off downhill. I'm like this is how I like to ride. Downhill is my sweet spot of cycling. Then there is the sharp right turn. There is a party tent to my left with a DJ. The crowd support is awesome. The neighbors are so encouraging. I start to notice a slight incline. Then I remember there is a hill coming up. Last year I wasn't ready for this hill and was having technical difficulties with my gears. I was ready this time. I was already in my lowest gear ready to take on THE HILL. I pedal and pedal through this hill. I don't stop. I am sweating from the humidity like a sinner in church. I make it to the top. HALLELUJAH. I can feel how dry my throat is, not good. I am on flat surface, I attempt the unimaginable I reach for my water bottle and lo and behold I reach it, drink some water and by a straight miracle from God I could put the bottle back in its holder. This is a huge feat. Go me Go me!!! I make the last right turn onto the loop and head to the end. I'm thinking I can do another loop. I keep going and make my 2nd loop. I'm thinking to myself I didn't even do this last year. I make it up THE HILL again. I reach for water again. I'm checking out the neighborhood. These folks are partying it up. I'm slightly hating because I wish I was out there chilling with a food truck or margaritas. After I make the right turn and head back to the finish, my lower back tells me that I should go ahead and make my exit. I head to the exit. I check RunKeeper and see I am short of 6 miles. I ride around the parking lot to make it an even 6 miles. I head back to our spot. 2 loops done. Now it's time to eat. Did I mention Angela and I smelled the grill as we headed out and it was hard to dismiss the smell and go for a ride. I'm back in the tent drinking water. Hydration is so necessary. I head over to dinner with some of my charlotte sisters. Dinner is delicious. Hamburger, pasta salad and ice-cold Coca-Cola and cookies. After dinner, head back over to the tent. I rest up for a bit. Then I head back out for my 2nd round. I have concluded that 2 loops really work for me. I get 2 more loops in. I am currently at 4 loops which puts me at 12 miles. I'm close to being at the halfway point of my goal. I have doubled last year total mileage. Lazy Johanna was at booty last year. I just enjoyed the event wasn't really interested in any goal. I do know I was hydrating properly because I was peeing like a person with a weak bladder. Kristina told me that is a good sign. That means that I am drinking enough fluids. If you are not peeing, then you should be worried. Good to know. I think I knew that but I pretty much live in my bathroom at home.

There is a midnight pizza party. We all head over to the pizza party. As I have burned some calories I devour the 2 slices of pizza that we are told to is the initial serving. Then you can come back for me. After eating the 2 slices I didn't even think about coming back for more. I head back to the tent to let my food settle. I decide to go back out for another round. Can you believe it's still hot as hades at 1am? Mother nature must be fighting with Bae again. At this point it is pitch black on the loop, I have my lights on full blast. There are some serious dark pockets out there. As I riding there are still some spectators on the course. I'm like do these folks don't go to bed around here. As I pedal up the hill, there are some dark spots and my paranoid self thinks what if someone jumps out at me. I've seen way too many horror movies. I finish my 3rd round. I am now at 18 miles. I've done 3 times I did last year, I come back to the tent. I hydrate a little. It's about 2:30am. I go lay down on my air mattress. I forgot the blanket in my trunk. I am so not going to get at this hour. I improvise and use my towel. I'm tossing and turning on my air mattress. My roommate in the Taj Mahal tent is the lovely Dawn Davis Calhoun. She's already out like a fat kid in dodgeball. I finally pass out. I wake up in what seems like 5 minutes later. I hear Kristina say she's going to get 1 more loop in before the sun comes up. I attempt to lift off the air mattress. If you could have seen me get off that thing you would have died laughing it was so funny. I finally get to my feet feeling like I just drank all night. I get my socks and clips on. I load up my bottles. I have 7 miles left to goal. Its nice out. Temperature has finally cooled off some. I knock these 2 loops out. There are a lot of runners out on the loop on the sidewalk. I see a few BGR ladies I'm assuming. They yell you "go get it sister girl" I smile back. I finish round 4. I'm under 25 miles. I roll past the ladies and tell them I have 1 mile to go and its way too much to go get another loop in, I'm just going to ride around the area. I ride up and down the street

and through the expo area and back in the parking lot. Run Keeper and my cat eye are

not seeing eye to eye. Cat Eye is off my .22 miles. I keep riding until the cat eye hits

25 miles. When it does I start to swell up a little because I have met my goal. I can go

buy the mileage sticker and add it to the collection. I head back to the tent. I can now

go eat breakfast. My work here is done. Later booty, Jo is done!!

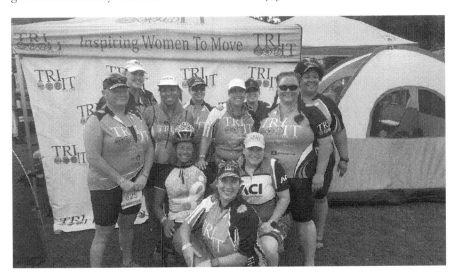

Rock 'N Roll Virginia Beach

September 4, 2016

Virginia Beach, Virginia

Rock N Roll marathon series sends out emails for all their upcoming races to their past race participants. I saw an email a few months ago, about Virginia Beach. I saw the medals and was hook, line and sinker. I went ahead and signed up. Few weeks later I started looking for hotels. It did not dawn on me that the hotel prices would be sky high. I reached out to my TRI sister Sharon Johnson who I knew had done the race previously. She reminded that the prices are $$$ and they run about $200-$300. I kept chastising myself for not checking hotel prices before I signed up. What's done is done. I eventually book a reasonably priced hotel in Norfolk per google maps it was about 15-minute drive from the race start.

I was rolling solo for this race. I tried to persuade my partner in crime, my mother, into signing up but she turned me down. Tall drink and his crew were signed up for the half. There was going to be a few familiar faces at the race.

Rock N Roll sent an email about the remix challenge. They offer a Saturday race, mile in the sand. If you do the Saturday race along with any other distance on Sunday you get the remix challenge medal, that makes a total of 3 medals. If you know me I LOVE bling and I cannot lie. I sign up for the mile in the sand. 3 medals coming up!!

I travel to Virginia Beach Friday afternoon. As I arrive at packet pickup, I check my phone and see a weather update from the race indicating the mile on the sand has been cancelled. Shocked but not disappointed. Hurricane Hermine is headed towards the east coast and she means business. I am at the race bib line, volunteer tells me about the race being cancelled but I will still pick up my medal and beach towel further down the hall. Race is cancelled but I still get my medal, beach towel SCORE!! I head to the 5K line, once I get to the counter the volunteer asks if I was signed up for Saturday's race. I respond yes and she gives me a black wristband that I will need to pick up my remix challenge medal on Sunday. Did I mention since Saturday's race is cancelled, they are giving us refunds? Won't he, do it? Will he won't? I prepaid for a parking pass and stop by and pick it up. Volunteer tells me I must be parked no later than 5:30am. My mouth hits the ground. I need to go to bed STAT. I've picked up all my stuff and head to my hotel.

Fast forward to Sunday morning. It's race day. My alarm goes off at 4am. I'm about a 19-minute drive from the convention center. I figure I would leave about 4:45 just to give myself extra time. I arrive at the convention center about 5am. I am not alone. The other early birds are there as well in FORMATION. After I park I have 2 hours until the race starts. A part of me is thinking if need be I could get a quick nap in but I know how much I enjoy my sleep so I stay awake listening to the radio. At 6am, my bladder tells me it needs to be emptied. I finally leave the comfort of my car. I head over to the porta potties and take care of business. I head over to my corral, #15. People are slowly showing up and lining up in the corrals. I meet a lady in my corral who is a local. She has done this race before but has gotten injured and been sidelined for a while and this race is her way to get back into the race game.

As we are waiting, another Half Fanatic asks me to take her picture. Turns out she is a BGR runner from Greensboro. I tell her I'm from Raleigh. Like one of my TRI sisters told me back at 24 HOB in Charlotte, "Jo you don't have a problem making friends". I really don't. Tall drink and his crew show up.

This is Shawnell's 2nd half. This is Donna's 1st half. I tell her she looks sleepy. She is. I told her you're here now. Too late to turn back the race starts at 7am. Since we are in corral #15, it's about 7:30 before we cross the start line. Once we do, I start my Garmin. This is his first race. The race starts in front of the convention center on 19th street and we head towards the oceanfront, just like Surf N Santa 5 miler in December except is not 40 degrees outside and it's not 5:30pm in the evening. I head out and I can tell I'm moving fast because my Garmin is reading 17:00/mile pace. Holy smokes batman!! I haven't seen that pace in about 3 years. I'm going to assume the Garmin is playing with me. After a while it reads my normal 20:00/mile pace. I try to not concentrate at looking at my watch. I'm listening to my music and moving. We make the first right. This is Rock N Roll race so there should be music. We make a left turn. We go about a block. we make another left and pass a church. They have a group singing. We are at mile 1. The Garmin vibrates and shows me my pace it's 20 minutes and some change. I'm thinking to myself the treadmill workouts have been paying out. Shout out to my trainer Gregory Clanton AKA Tall drink who has been pushing me. We make a right turn and another right onto Atlantic avenue. As we do I see the hotel my mom and I stayed in back in March for Shamrock. I'm thinking oh so we will not be finishing by King Neptune, BUMMER! King Neptune is a must-see attraction at Virginia Beach.

We are headed down Atlantic, finally pass the water stop. Thank you to all the volunteers. Without you, races would not happen. I can see in the distance the 5K turn. I look and it's the same turn for Surf N Santa right by the hotel Angel Chappell Jones and I stayed at back in December. It's obvious I've been up here a lot for races. There was no mistake that I was going to miss the 5K turn because adding an extra 10 miles is not part of my plan. I make the left turn onto the boardwalk. I see runners already on the boardwalk. SHUT THE FRONT DOOR!! There are folks finishing the half already. The fast folks started earlier so that makes sense but it still boggles my mind these folks are finishing 13.1 miles in 90 minutes. Let's take a minute and do the math. Per my calculations that's about a 6.87 minute/pace. I can't even imagine. Hats off to those speed demons!! That's BQ qualifying time. I'm on the boardwalk which is full of spectators on the sidelines cheering. I cross the finish line and the time clock reads 1:31 minutes. I know that's not my time the race clock time. I stop my Garmin for some bizarre reason that sucker wants to keep going. It takes me 2 good tries to finally get it to stop. Need to read up on the proper stop/start process. I'm given my 5K medal. One of the medical teams comes up to me and ask I'm ok. Maybe I looked like I needed help. I told her I'm fine. I'm going to try to not read anything into that. She was doing her job. Where is my side eye emoji???

After I receive my medal, volunteers are passing out water, Gatorade. I lost count on how many times my picture was taken. I enjoy the RNR races but I must tell you they need to step up their post-race refreshment. I have probably gotten spoiled by races that have pizza, barbecue sandwiches, Irish stew. Yep I have gotten spoiled. A slice of pizza would have hit the spot. I ask a volunteer as I exit the finish line area where do I pick up my remix challenge medal and he points to a table further up the boardwalk. I head over and I hear a volunteer explain to someone that you had to have signed up for the Saturday race to get it. As I walk over and show my black wristband, she tells the person "this lady LOVES to run" No I love the bling!! Rock N Roll VB is in the books.

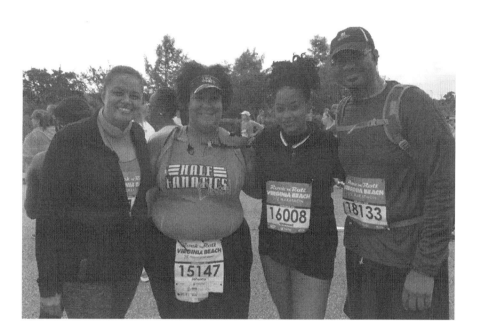

Wicked 10K & Monster Mile

October 29, 2016

Virginia Beach, Virginia

I have become a serious fan of J&A racing. They sponsor the Coastal Virginia Running series. I have had the pleasure of participating in 3 out of the 7 events. I've been a repeat customer of 1 of their events, the awesome fabulous Yuengling Shamrock half marathon and 8K AKA as the dolphin challenge. Come join me next year! Registration is currently open. Didn't I mention I was a fan :-) They sponsor Anthem Wicked 10K which is a Halloween themed race along with the historic monster mile. The 2 races happen about 2.5 hours apart. Therein lies the real challenge.

It dawned on me as we were preparing to head on our journey. This is the 3rd time I've been to Virginia Beach for a race this year. I really must like it there. Shamrock in March, Rock N Roll in September and now Wicked.

My partner in crime, Angel Chappell Jonas, drove up from Charlotte. Then we headed to Virginia Beach from Raleigh. Dynamic duo is back at it. Reunited and it feels so good. We head to the race expo when we get there. I really enjoy race expos. I'm like a kid in a candy store. As we walked in, I noticed the expo was in a smaller space than Shamrock. Angel told me it was in the same place it was last year. I was explaining that the entrance for Shamrock expo was further down because the course maps were on display on wall monitors. I can describe every detail of Shamrock expo. It's my favorite of all race expos. We pick up our packets and get our IDs checked for the beer tent. I'm probably the one runner/walker/racer that I know that's not a beer drinker. I typically will try at least 1 beer after the race. Blue Moon is one of the race sponsors. Just about ALL the beer drinkers I know rave about Blue Moon. After we peruse through all the vendors, we head over to our hotel and check in. The 2nd most exciting thing about this weekend is the absolute awesome rate for this hotel. The cost for the 1 room for the weekend = the cost for 1 night at the Hilton resort which is right next door and where I have been completely obsessed with staying since I first saw it. You can't beat that with a stick. As we are checking into the hotel, brother working at the front desk kills my dream and tells me that I would be disappointed if I stayed at the Hilton. I think he tells me this because it is their direct competition. He tells me that's what he does kill folks dream and laughs it off. You never know who you going to meet. Angel told me later that dude was flirting with me. I totally missed that since he killed my Hilton dream. Any who dude had to be old enough to be my dad. In the words of Quentin Snively "Jo you need an older southern gentleman" in your life.

Race is Saturday morning. 10K starts at 8am. Monster mile starts at 10:30am. Race start is at the convention center which per google is a good 1.5 miles from our hotel. Lazy Johanna thinks we should just take an Uber to the race start. I'm outvoted by Angel who tells me will walk along with other racers who will be walking. We head out a little after 7am and make our TREK to the convention center. It's about 40ish degrees outside. We have plastic trash bags on to keep us warm. The downside to this is keeps the heat inside which makes "premenopausal" Johanna heat up very fast. I'm sweating like a sinner in church and we haven't even started the race yet. By the time, we get to the race start, I am hot and sweaty like I have finished the race. This was sign #1 of my issue that I did not address. We head to our corral which is the last one. Because I am slightly concerned about my finish time to be back for the monster mile, we go out with an early corral. It's our corral's turn to head to the start line. We cross the start line and off we go. Garmin is set and we head out. I'm a walker but there are runners flying past me like they are in the Indy 500. Let's just with the fast folks rolling past me I've gotten out in a faster pace than I normally do. This is issue #2, going too fast out the gate. I went totally against my own rule, your race your pace. Angel and I are moving along. As we leave the convention center, I tell Angel this route is just like Rock N Roll which I just did Labor Day weekend and Surf N Santa which we did back in December. We make a right onto Atlantic. We go all the way down Atlantic and come up onto the boardwalk at the end. The weather is nice and the wind is nowhere as heavy as it was back in March when we turned onto the boardwalk for Shamrock 8K. We turn off the boardwalk and back onto Atlantic. We pass the 5K point. The race clock is at hour and some change. It will be another hour plus before I finish. I mention to Angel about the time. She reminds me we must be lined up by 10:30 for the mile. I tell her at the rate I'm going I'm not going to make it to the mile race. I tell her to go on and to not let me hold her back. She heads off. Did I mention there is a zombie zone at the 5K mark? I'm still raw from the season premiere of TWD. I ain't got no time for no zombie zone. My 5K time is about 68 minutes which is more than what I have been doing on the treadmill. I tell myself no worries, we are out here to get this race done. I'm really starting to feel warm from sweating and I'm starting to rethink the long running pants I decided to wear. As I am coming up Atlantic wouldn't you know I pass our hotel. I see the Max sitting in the parking lot. I contemplate for a minute of taking a detour and heading up the room. That isn't a realistic option because that will not get me the 6.2 miles I need and it won't get me the medal either. I tell Lazy Johanna we are not tapping out. I keep moving forward. I'm wondering when are we going to turn on to the boardwalk. I realize the turn on to the boardwalk is the same as it is for Shamrock just in the opposite direction. I turn right onto the boardwalk entrance. There is an aid station with Krispy Kreme doughnuts. volunteer ask me if I want small or large doughnut. I'm so out of it. I tell the volunteer don't make me must make a real decision. She gives me the small. Doughnut tastes good. A few yards after eating the doughnut my throat is dry from the sugar. I take a sip on my Camelback and keep moving. I'm on the boardwalk and I don't see the finish line. I'm like when is this thing going to end. I pass a water stop at mile 5. Bunch of teenagers working this water stop. they high five me as I pass them. One of them is dressed as Hillary Clinton which is hilarious because it's a guy. I grab some water and keep moving. I glance out at the Atlantic Ocean and really is gorgeous out there. I have 1.2 miles left to go to the finish. I think I can I think I can. These 2 guys are walking out on the boardwalk. They ask me if I'm going to be alright. I mumble yeah. When you are hot and headed towards dehydration you really don't have a lot to say. They pass me as they head down the boardwalk. I keep walking. I hear a noise coming up beside me. It's a race vehicle on a golf cart. One of the guys ask me "are you doing the race" Smart ass Johanna really wanted to say, "what the HELL do you think I'm out here doing" I kept it PC and told them yes. I guess they were out looking for any participants still on the course. I shall call them the sweepers because they pretty much tailed me the rest of the way.

My pace is getting slower and slower. I glance at my Garmin and it is reading 27 minutes. At this point I don't care I just want to be done. I pass a lady sitting on a bench. She tells me "you're doing better than me I can't even do what you're doing so keep it up" Words from a stranger can give you just a slight boost of energy you need to get you where you need to go. I keep on walking. I can start to see the finish line in the distance. Guess who I pass on a bench taking a rest, the 2 dudes who asked me earlier if I was ok. I ask them "what are you doing sitting down" They just start laughing. 1 of the guys catches up to me and tells me that his friend has had hip surgery and had both knees replaced. He's glad that he can get him out and about moving. No idea why this random stranger felt to tell me his friend's life story but it got my mind off how tired I was feeling. Thank you, random dude, on the boardwalk! I pass King Neptune. There are 2 cops nearby and they tell me "you are almost there" I respond back "I actually believe you" I spy with my little eye the finish line banner and the tents. I keep moving because I know I got this. Suddenly I hear a police siren. I see the police on the motorcycle. then it dawns on me that the monster mile first finisher is coming through. Then I see another motorcycle cop and then I see the kids running. They are running like the wind headed to the finish line. Seeing these kids pass me would probably mess with someone else it really gave me life. I'm heading into the finish arch which has these ghost decorations hanging from it. I hear the announcer calling names and I hear him call my name that was all I needed to get me to the finish. I cross the finish line and I've never been so glad to be done with a race in my life. I head through the finish line chute to get to the medals. All I see are the mile medals. One of the volunteers sees my 10K bib and heads over to get me one.

Then I ask about the mile medal. I show them my 2nd bib and they give me the mile medal. Technically I didn't do the monster mile but do you think I care. I sure don't. I'm going to count the 1.5 pre-race mile towards that race. A volunteer passes me a water bottle. I find a spot on a bench and I am so glad to sit down that I really don't think I will be able to get up anytime soon.

Since the mile finishers are coming in, I decide I will wait for Angel to come in. Literally like 5 minutes later, I see her coming through the finish line chute and wave to her. She tells me I need to get on up and keep moving. It really takes me a few minutes to tell my body that we are going to get up off the bench. I finally get up and I am hobbling through the finish line chute. My right foot is feeling funky and I'm just dead tired. I ask Angel where did you get the finisher hat. She tells me it's almost at the end. We head there and I get my hat. At this point, I don't even care about the soup and beer that's waiting on the beach. Angel can see that I don't look so good so she forces me to go get some soup. I hobble onto the beach into the sand which is a real struggle. Angel tells the soup tent is right there. I'm so glad because there's no way I could go any further. I get the tomato and cheese soup and bread. I tell Angel I'm headed over to the benches by Dairy Queen. She heads to the beer tent. I could care less about the beer even though I wanted to try Blue Moon. Not today.

The finish line is at 19th street. Our hotel is at 30th street. That's about 11 blocks to get back to the hotel. I tell Angel why don't we just call an Uber. She tells me the Uber driver will laugh at us from taking a ride from the finish line. I'm like SO!! We start walking to the hotel on the bike path. My feet are hurting. My lower back has started talking to me. I pull out my phone and order a Lyft ride. I'm a Lyft girl primarily because I used to drive for them.

I tell Angel to go right ahead and keep walking back to the hotel but I just ordered a ride and I'm going to wait for them to get here. She keeps on going. I get into my Lyft ride. My Lyft driver is Kenneth. I tell him he is a godsend. He tells me that sounds like a $30 tip. Slow your horse's sir giving him serious side eye. When he drops me off at my hotel I do give him a nice tip because he just saved my life by giving me a ride. Thank you, Kenneth, my Lyft driver!

Wicked 10K is done. I've learned that I need to stop being hard headed and refuel properly during the race. I need to dress for how warm it will be and not how cold it starts out. With all that being said, I'm very glad that I persevered and made it to finish line. I have no doubt that I will finish Richmond on November 12 with my mom by my side.

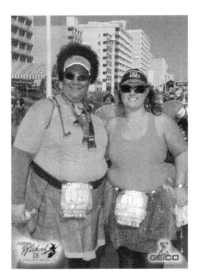

American Family Fitness Half Marathon

Richmond, Virginia

November 12, 2016

I participated in the Richmond half marathon for the first time in 2015. A few days after finishing the race, I signed up for the 2016 race primarily because I was pretty much hooked on this race due to the finisher swag they give out. They offered a sweet race registration price of $60. The same registration deal is currently active right now for the 2017 race. I'll save you some time and tell you that I will be signing up before the deal ends on the 17th.

My mom has drunk the Kool-Aid along with the rest of us. She was signed up for the race as well. She flew up to Raleigh on Thursday. We drove up to Richmond on Friday. We headed straight to the race expo after making a pit stop at Cracker Barrel.

My partner in crime AKA my trainer AKA my personal drill sergeant AKA tall drink was already at the expo waiting on us. We met up with him at the expo. We made the rounds after picking up our shirt and bib.

141

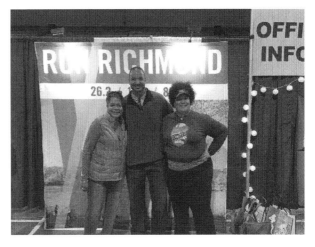

While perusing the various vendors at the expo, we run into the Click It Hot booth. I see the same guy that I have run into at the last 3 races. He recognizes me. He tells mom and tall drink about their products. I am already a fan as I bought the handheld pads about 2 weeks at the Wicked expo. He persuades my mom in buying the large pad. I mention how I left mine in the fridge at home. He gives me one for free and my mom one as well. Thank you very kindly. I highly recommend them.

After we finish up at the expo, we go check into the hotel, hit the pasta buffet at the hotel. That buffet was on point. Pasta, salad, and dessert. Shout out to Crowne Plaza for providing all the hotel guests doing the race with a bag of free goodies including banana, bottle of water and granola bar. Breakfast is served and we didn't have to make a grocery store run.

Saturday morning shows up in like 5 minutes. Mom and I head out and make the 5-block trek to the start line which really feels so much longer. It's a cold 35 degrees outside. I'm cold natured so I have lost count on how many layers I have on.

I'm that one person who does not throw away her layers. My clothes cost $$ and they are going back home with me. We head to corral K which is at the back of the bus literally. The wind is blowing which is making it feel so much colder. We notice folks are huddled in the archway of buildings to block the wind, very smart. I meet a fellow BGR lady who is doing the race as well. This is her 1st half marathon. I remember what that is like. She asks me what my game plan is, in other words, am I doing intervals? If so what are they. Probably for the last few years I don't have a race game plan, I just show up and put 1 foot in front of the other and do my best to not be carried out on a stretcher. A few of my TIFL sisters are doing the race as well. They find me and mom in the corral. Shout out to the TRI tribe who was at Richmond, Monica Oliver, Ebony Haywood, Cynthia Gary and Kathy Beasley.

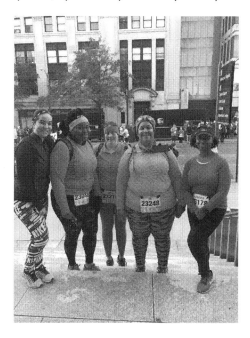

Ebony tells me "Jo is that tall drink from the blog?" I tell her yeah and have you seen him. She tells me he was waiting on some corner. I later tell tall drink that he's blog famous ☺

The race starts at 7:30am. We line up in the corral and move towards the start line as the corrals are released out onto the course. Our corral crosses the start line about 12 minutes after the start. I start the Garmin and off we go. The race goes down Broad street in downtown Richmond. Mom, myself and tall drink are walking together. Mom decides to pick up her pace and moves further ahead of us. I tend to get into a weird zone during a race. I'm not real talkative. I'm really inside my head contemplating why I even sign up for this torture. It's an internal debate that happens during every race. Tall drink keeps checking on me which is a good thing. You never know if my body has decided to tap out. We pass mile 2 and there is a water stop and bathroom. Potty pit stop, yes please!! Pit stop is complete, we keep going. We come up on the turn. The cops are there directing folks. Marathon goes left. Half marathon goes right. I knew where we were going. I told tall drink missing your turn and being on the marathon course is not a mistake you want to make. We turn right. I know we are headed towards the baseball stadium which is the home of the flying squirrels. I passed their booth at the race expo, that's how I know the team name. There is an aid station outside the stadium. They have music playing. I tell tall drink you see my mom down there. They are playing Michael Jackson and my mom is dancing up a storm. My mom is having a ball. We pass the stadium. I mention to tall drink that this is where the race expo was held the day before. We go under I-95 and head into a neighborhood. We turn right into the neighborhood and there is a loop and then we come out the neighborhood. I start noticing the names of the streets, Robin Hood,

144

Sherwood Forest. I'm like was Robin Hood from Richmond. I must google this later. We are out the neighborhood and make on the main street. Suddenly I hear a car coming, I'm thinking here comes the 1st marathon finisher. Then we hear the bike leads yell out "marathon finisher" Tall drink ask me about it. I tell him that is the 1st marathon finisher passing us. Soon after we see more marathoners passing us. YES, the marathoners are coming!! They are flying like the wind bullseye. I'm starting to feel a little hunger coming on. I reach out for a granola bar. I unwrap it and wouldn't you know 2/3 of the bar fall on the ground. That hurt me to my core. Tall drink tells you are not picking that up. I really wanted to and ask for God to bless it. I was outvoted. I eat what's left of my granola bar and keep it moving. We head towards the half marathon turn into the park. This is where I lost the course last year. Good times. As we go into the park, there is a partition up and I see other half marathoners coming out the park. I see 2 of my tri sisters, Cynthia and Kathy. Folks are giving me High-Fives. Amazing how such a small gesture can give you a major boost of energy. It really did. We are in the park and it must run past I-95 because you can see cars on the highway. We are moving through the park and we pass the 6-mile mark and the timing mat. I'm really starting to feel overheated and dehydrated. Pretty much the same way I felt at this same mile marker a year ago. I stop and if tall drink wasn't standing by me I probably would have hit the ground. I drink some water and work on getting my breathing under control. The SAG car is behind us. My mom walks up to him and tells him I'm not doing so good. He pulls up and I am told to get in. I get in and we drive further up on the course. I tell the cop about being out here last year and getting lost. GUESS WHAT!!! He tells me that was him. I'm like hey buddy!! This

145

POWER OF THE TURTLE:TALES OF BEING DEAD LAST

is the same cop who got lost with me last year. It's a small world after all. As we pass course monitors through the park, he lets them know there are still folks on the course. Last year, them rascals hauled tail and left their post too early. You see I'm still bitter about that a whole year later. We find the turn we missed last year. No way on God's green earth we would have seen it last year. We make our way out the park and back to the turn. I get out and get back on the course. I'm feeling so much better. I stop at the aid station and get something of everything they have. I've been sweating so I know I need to replenish my fluids. Of course, the Garmin is all confused about the mileage because I didn't stop it when I got in the car. Oh well. Per, the course I am at mile 8, I have 5.1 miles left to go. HALLELUJAH!! This part of the course is fun primarily because the neighborhoods go all out. They have unofficial aid stations through here with Coca-Cola, beer, candy, chips. You name it. I pass on the beer. I take some of the candy. Tall drink calls to check up on me, I tell him I'm doing ok. He tells me they will catch up with me shortly. I keep putting 1 foot in front of the other. Soon I am out of the neighborhood and I am on a main street. I turn right and I pass the campus of Virginia Union University #HBCULove. I remember passing here last year and I was really struggling. I was talking to tall drink on the phone for motivation. Then I heard an angel whose name is Kat Collier yell out my name. Her energy gave me life. She was like "jo we only have 2 miles left to go". I want to get some of that energy the marathoners have. I'm working on getting there. I pass VUU. Marathoners are on the left. Half marathoners are on the right. Suddenly someone runs up to me, guess who it is, 1 of my TRI sisters Miya Caswell who is doing the marathon.

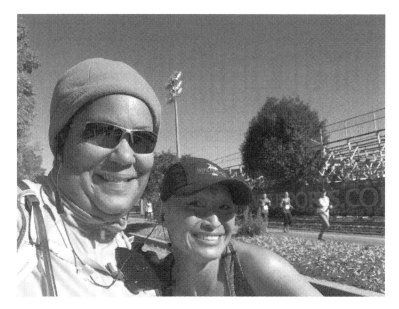

She tells me later that seeing me energized her to get to the finish line. That's exactly what she did for me. She takes off running back on the marathon side. A few minutes later, guess who walks up to me up out of the blue, tall drink. I'm like where is my mom. He points behind us and there is my mom heading towards us. My mom who is 65 years old is coming on down the course doing her 2nd half marathon. Did you hear me??

My 65-year old mother is doing a half marathon. Yes, my mom is better than yours!! The 3 of us are back together on the course. We head up another hill. Tall drink asks me if there are any more. I tell him I don't remember all these hills. We are coming back into downtown. We cross over Broad street. We turn left, there is this group out cheering. I'm going to say they may have been intoxicated because they were loud. I could be mistaken. The red solo cups could prove I was right. They were

147

giving out High-Fives which I was getting some of. High-fives = super energy power when you are out on the race course. I really know that we don't have that much further to go. We pass through Virginia Commonwealth University campus AGAIN. I know we are getting close. I see a lady come up to us. She asks me if I did the race last year. Guess who it is? The run coach who I met last year who thought it was my first race and I decided to mess with her and tell her I had done the dolphin challenge back in March at Virginia Beach. Don't let the fluff fool you? I get in my miles just like everyone else. She tells me she just met my mom who came all the way from Alabama. I'm like yeah that's my mom. She tells me that I'm doing better than last year. Last year it was much later when she saw me. I was oblivious to how much time had passed on the course. I never know. I wear a Garmin. We are going through downtown streets. Folks are telling us we only have a few more turns left. I know for a fact that we do. We make the last left turn. I tell tall drink that we are headed to the finish. I tell him to look ahead and he sees the downhill finish. I hear a group of folks yell my name and it's some of my nOg & Galloway peeps who have finished the race and headed out. We are coming down the hill. I tell tall drink we just passed my hotel. I tell him that's just disrespectful that I'm passing right by my hotel but I can't go in yet. We go down the hill and I hear the announcer call our names. We cross the finish line. Thank God, I made it to the finish line. Half marathon #10 is done.

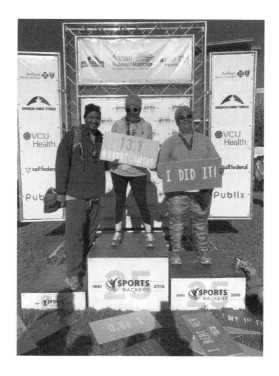

Jingle Bell Run Raleigh 5K

December 3, 2016

Raleigh, NC

I like participating in local races. Jingle bell run is a Christmas themed race that supports the Arthritis foundation.

Folks really get into dressing up. I've been participating in this race for at least 5 years that I can recall. I love the race shirts they are so festive. I feel deep down in my spirit that the race could use a finisher's medal. I'm just saying. Then again, I am a medal chick. A nice Christmas medal would look good on the medal rack. I shall send them an email with my suggestion.

The race started at 10:30am. The race is held at Saint Mary's School. There is no parking on campus. I knew the parking would be limited. I left the house with the goal of being parked before 9am. As I turned onto the side street by the school, I could tell that I was not the only one who was getting there early. I turned onto the 1st side street by the school and found a parking spot, I spy with my little eye one of my TRI sisters and running buddies Lille Thompson-Ebron. As we start walking towards the race headquarters, I run into one of my NCRC buddies Terri Saylor. We made our way to the entrance of Saint Mary's. I mention to Lillie and Terri that the race registration used to be in the cafeteria where we could use the indoor restroom facilities which is a big difference from the portable facilities. I feel that something has happened that has now required the race to be completed outside. That's my inner conspiracy theorist coming out.

As we are at the entrance of Saint Mary's, we look for a sunny spot to warm up in while we wait for the race start. We are super-duper early for the race. As we are waiting around, I see my partner in crime Melanie Shaw walking towards me.

She told me that I am the reason she started walking and doing 5Ks about a year ago. It always amazes me when someone tells me that because I never really think about that when I am out doing races. I just do them primarily for the exercise and the medals. What can I tell you I like bling and I cannot lie? Melanie tells me she has met some new friends. We are friendly people. We met folks everywhere we go.

My bladder has been acting nervous all morning. I make a beeline for the outdoor facilities. We go and hang out with the new peeps over on a bleacher in the sun near the entrance. As I walk back I hear someone call my name. It's Debbie

150

Hockstra, one of my former NCRC Women's beginner running peeps. She tells me that is so motivated to see me doing races and she bets there are others who are if they aren't already. She tells me that folks should realize that a race is possible instead of thinking that it isn't. I tell her about Melanie. She says that's what I'm talking about. You motivate folks and you don't even realize it. True I really don't.

Another 1 of my TRI sisters Cynthia Gary meets up with us. We keep running into more of the TRI tribe, Kathy Beasley and Patty Cooper, Renee Weinchinger and Valerie McGlynn and Beth Griffin and finally Meredith Cuomo. TIFL reunited and it feels so good.

The 1 mile starts at 10am. Lillie asks me if I want to switch from the 5K. she's funny. I do like a 1-mile race, easy peasy. We go line up after the one mile starts. We are passing the corrals. 8-10-minute mile, 10-12-minute mile. I tell Lillie that is so far off from where I am. She says Jo if you get back to running you could get there. I tell her I really want to get to a consistent 18:00/mile pace. That is my goal that I have set for myself. We head to the last corral which is 15 minute/strollers & walkers. Melanie asked me "Does that say 15 minutes to do a mile?" I tell her yes but it also says walkers and that's what we are. We head to the back of the corral and wait for the race start. 10:30 has come and gone. We are starting to get antsy. We look up and see folks moving and we head to the start. I tell Cynthia I'm not starting my Garmin until we cross the timing mat. We cross the timing mat and I start the Garmin and RunKeeper. I'm also signed up for 2 5K challenges on RunKeeper, might as well kill 2 birds with 1 stone. We head down Hillsborough street. In case you are not aware, Hillsborough street is HILLY. We are up and down the street. We come up on the

Alexander YMCA and across the street is a guy in full attire playing the bagpipes. I recognize him from afar, it's Ashby Spratley, my former honey badger group pace leader from Galloway. As we are walking I meet a lady who's name I didn't get it until we were almost done lol. As we are walking and talking, I find out she has done triathlons. Isn't that a coinky dink. Get this she has done open water triathlon. I tell her that she is officially badass because I like the pool and I cannot lie. She did Outer Banks triathlon back in September and she did not train. Double badass. Who in the world does an open water tri and does not train?? This badass lady. She tells me that she injured herself by running on the beach. She has had a knee brace on ever since and is wearing it right now. She wanted to do the race because she had committed to so her and the knee brace made the race. AMAZING!! We are walking and talking, before we know it we have passed the 1-mile mark. I hear a kid behind me tell his mom "we've only gone 1 mile" Bless their heart. I notice there is a lot of development on Hillsborough Street. Its apparent I have not been on this end in a long time. I see one my FAV Galloway peeps Meri Kotlas who is a course monitor. She high-five's me. This is probably the 1st race in a long time that I'm enjoying the race, course and just having a good time. That's exactly what tall drink told me to do today, have fun and enjoy the race. I can see ahead that we are getting close to the turnaround, woo hoo!! As we get closer I notice this new building with stores and restaurants below it. I'm like there's the new Pieology place that my movie peeps were talking about the other night. Then I see an IHOP. I'm thinking so that's why they closed the other one down. Melanie asks me where is the turnaround and I tell her it's right by the cop car. We all make the turnaround and head back to the finish. The pace car has been tailing

152

us the whole time. Cynthia told me at the start that I like having a cop tail me. She's

funny. I tell her it's important that they are back there just in case something happens.

I have needed them both times I've done Richmond. Thank you, Raleigh PD, for

being out there with us turtles today!! As we are heading back, the cop tells the course

monitors they are done. They start walking back with us. We pass Meri and she joins

us. As we pass other corners, she lets course monitors know they are done. We pick

up more course monitors. Meri calls it a course monitor parade. I tell my new friend

whose name is Laura that we are passing the bell tower, major landmark down. Right

before we passed the bell tower, volunteers are holding up the 2-mile marker signs.

They tell us we have 1 mile left to go. We pass the traffic circle right by the bell tower.

We pass the doubletree hotel. Meri mentions that Ashby was out here. We both

wonder if he still is. We don't see him. We pass by the YMCA again. I know we are

getting close to the finish. We pass Ashe avenue which leads to Pullen Park. We are

almost there. Since I know the route I know we really are. We pass another traffic

circle. We have an uphill finish. Isn't that nice? I look up and I see an angel coming to

me. I yell out EBONY!! It's 1 of my TRI sisters Ebony Haywood. She tells me I came

out to support you and see you finish the race. That's what I'm talking about.

Sisterhood and support. You can't buy this. No, you cannot. She tells me that I am

probably going to beat my Holly Springs time. I can see the time clock in the distance.

I see 68 minutes. I'm thinking we probably crossed a few minutes after that. Cynthia

and Lillie are right behind the finish. They are cheering me on as well. We cross over

the finish line. I stopped the Garmin and RunKeeper. Finish time 1:06:47 with a pace

of 21:02/mile. My treadmill workouts have been paying off. Jingle Bell Run is in the books.

Suggly Sweater 5K

December 17, 2016

Holly Springs, NC

Suggly Sweater 5K is my last race of 2016. I looked back over my list of races for this year and this was my 10th 5K. Holy Smokes batman I have been doing a lot of races. Who knew? I did because I keep a running list so I know what I have coming up and what I have done. I won't even mention the half marathons, 10K, 8K and triathlons. This has been a busy year for me in terms of races. I'm blessed to have been able to do it all. I'm looking forward to 2017 and everything that awaits me.

I saw an advertisement for the Suggly Sweater race at Omega Sports in Cary when I was picking up my race packet for Holly Spring 5K. What caught my attention was that it was a local 5K and there was a medal. If you know me, you know how I feel about medals. Shockingly I did not take a picture of the sign. After I got home I kept trying to rack my memory on what the name of the race was. To my own surprise and through the helpfulness of Google I could find it. Cost was $35 which wasn't too bad in my opinion. I went ahead and signed up. Of course, I decided to share the race on social media in case some of my fellow race peeps might be interested in joining me.

The race was held on December 17 at Sug Farm Park in holly Springs. I have lived in Wake county for over 18 years. There are still parts of it that I have never heard of. This gets added to the list. Raleigh is the capital of North Carolina and the major city in the county. There are others including Cary, Wake Forest, Apex, Holly

Springs and Fuquay-Varina. When I venture into the neighboring towns, it boggles me to see how much they have going on. When I drove to Holly Springs in November for the Inaugural half-marathon and 5K I was really impressed with the baseball stadium the race was held at. Who knew Holly Springs had it going on like that? I live in my corner of Northeast Raleigh and that's about it.

As I woke up on Saturday morning for the race, I check my phone and see there was slick road conditions overnight that caused serious crashes on the roads. I slowly go into panic mode. I wonder if the roads are safe and if I should just stay home and miss the race. I really don't want to miss the race primarily because it's my last race and it's the last race report I'm going to put in the book. SN: I'm working on a book about my race adventures. I text 2 of my TRI sisters Tiffany Davis and Ebony Haywood to see what they think. Neither responds. I call tall drink to see what he thinks. He isn't really fazed by the weather. I decided to go ahead and get ready and head down US-1 to Holly Springs. By the time, I get dressed and get my stuff together, Ebony texts me that she's in route to the race. Tiffany is barely among the wake. I head out on the TREK from my neck of the woods down to Holly Springs. It's a good 35-minute drive. I really must love races because I'm not about the commute life anymore. I head toward the park entrance and I can tell from the line of cars heading into the parking area that the weather is having absolutely no impact of the attendance. Folks are rolling in like normal. Did I mention that the temperature is a COLD 32 degrees outside? Baby it's cold outside. I'm really wondering why I didn't put on like 1 more layer just in case.

As I park in the parking area, I sit and wait in the car. I call tall drink. He can hear it in my voice that I'm not in a good race mode. My mind is all over the place thinking about other stuff. I tend to overstress over things. He reminds me to have a good race and have fun. I gather up my camelback and my phone and head over to the race HQ. The wind is kicking up and making the 32 degrees feel like 22 degrees. I'm starting to rethink doing races in December. Ebony and Kathy are already at the race sitting in Kathy's car. Claudia Mello is also at the race as well. I wait by the entrance to race HQ for them. I see Tiffany walking up. We walk around trying to stay warm. It really isn't working. We walk past a table that has a snow waiver that you can sign if you plan on using any of the snow shops that have set up. No thank you. We walk past 1 of the snow stations. They have ice shooting into a machine making real snow. The snow is COLD. I'll pass. Kids are enjoying it. I see a few heaters under one of the tents where folks are hovering around it to stay warm. I tell Tiffany it reminds me of Charleston 5K. She tells me it's just like Rock N Roll Raleigh. I tell her you know I wasn't there I sent my replacement. Kathy and Ebony finds us. We get a pre-race group picture. Then we head over to the start line.

The start of the race is in the field. I don't even remember hearing anyone saying GO. I look up and see folks in front of us take off. We start moving towards the start line and we all set our Garmin's once we cross the timing mat. GARMINS unite!! The race goes around the outer perimeter of the field. The terrain is very unbalanced and I'm trying my best not to fall because I am seriously accident prone just check out the mysterious bruises that show up on my arms and legs. I really can't tell you where they came from either. Maybe I'm in an imaginary abusive relationship with my bed that I don't know about. You got to admit that was funny. We are making our way around the field. As we go down the side of the field, Tiffany says what goes down must come up. Then we start to walk up the field. We make our way around the front side of the field. There are some signs and markings that tell us where to go. We pass around the start/finish line and head around the field again. Tiffany tells me the first finishers are already headed to the finish. Overachievers!! I mean that in complete love. We head back down the side of the field. There is a sign that says 2 and right. We turn right and we are on the trail again and then we pass mile 1 marker. Garmin beeps and mile 1 is at 21:51. I'll take it. We keep moving through the trail and have mercy we finally are on the greenway. Tiffany and I both rejoice that we are on solid ground. The trail was killing my feet and tearing up Tiffany's hip and knees. It's hard out here for the Aruba TRI queens (nickname that tall drink has given us since we are signed up to do Challenge Aruba in October 2017). The greenway is very desolate. There are no course monitors out there. Tiffany mentions what if I was out here by myself. This is the prime spot for a predator to attack. Well I be she is right. As just as soon as she said that we see 3 teenagers who are course monitors. I tell Tiffany she talked them up. They tell us to keep up the good work. After we pass them we finally see a water stop. We were wondering if there was any kind of support out here on this course. I take a water cup and its ice cold and feels good to my throat. I am sweating like a sinner in church. Even in 30-degree weather I am sweating. We pass the water stop and keep on pushing on. I tell Tiffany the greenway reminds me of the greenway in Cary where the commitment day race went on. The greenway is running behind new houses that are being built. It's hilly. We keep pushing through. We come to one hill. We both take a pause before we attack it. My lower back is starting to talk to me and not in a good way. My feet are doing very well. That's normally where my issues are. We make it up the hill. We are coming around the side of a field. We have passed mile marker 2 awhile back. As we head out the greenway, we see cop cars at the entrance. It dawns on me that we are headed back to the park entrance. That means we are almost done. We turn onto the street. We tell the cops we are the last ones on the course. We see cars leaving as we head to the finish. I hear someone yell "Jo". Guess who it is? Meredith Cuomo one of my TRI sisters. I didn't even know she was even out here doing the race. We keep walking towards the park. Some cars honk at us as they are leaving. Some folks are giving us virtual high 5s as we pass them. It's stuff like that gives me that extra boost of energy to keep on moving. My phone rings and its tall drink checking on us. I tell him we are headed to finish. Tiffany yells out we have .5 miles left to go. He tells me to call when we finish because he wants to know our time. SN: Tall drink has been designated our personal drill sergeant to get us ready for Aruba. We cross into the park and pass the parking area. I tell Tiffany this is the part that sucks when you pass by your car but you can't get it in just yet. As we get closer to the turn to the finish, I spy with my little eye 2 of our TRI sisters up ahead Ebony and Kathy. I would like to call them Ebony & Ivory but someone make think that's offensive. I tell Tiffany that's what I'm talking about, sisterhood and support. We turn onto the field and head to the finish line. I see another TRI sister on the side, Claudia Mello. She heads to the finish line and is taking pictures of us. We cross the finish line posing. We have finished the race.

It was so much better having someone with me this time. Thank you,

Tiffany Davis, for signing up and doing this race with me. Racing is so much fun with a friend.

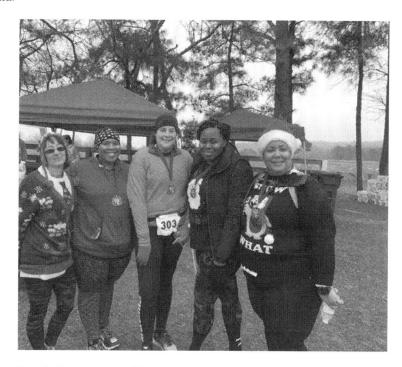

It really blows my mind how much I have done since I started on this athletic journey in 2008. Back when I signed up for the beginner running program, I had no idea what the future held for. There is a familiar saying that I've heard and I have used to folks who are hesitant about participating in a race, "you never know what you can until you try." This is a very true statement. Once you step out of your comfort zone, amazing things can happen.

ABOUT THE AUTHOR

Johanna Outlaw is an experienced athlete who wants to share her race experiences with men and women with hopes that it will inspire them to reach their health and wellness goals.

Johanna has worked in corporate America in the telecommunications industry for over 17 years. After being downsized in 2015 due to outsourcing, she has decided to pursue entrepreneurial opportunities by starting her own business, Healthy at Any Size.

She currently resides in Raleigh, North Carolina. In her free time, she mentors future triathletes, volunteers at local races, enjoys movies, reading books and listening to music.

90506704R00089

Made in the USA
Columbia, SC
08 March 2018